Who's in Control
of your Multiple Sclerosis?

Pieces of the MS Recovery Puzzle

WILLIAM E. CODE, MD, FRCPC (Anesthesiology)
DENISE CODE, Msc (Nutrition), RD

Who's in Control
of your Multiple Sclerosis?

WORDS
·OF·
WISDOM
PRESS

ISBN 0-9737918-0-2
ISBN 978-0973-7918-0-8

Printed in Canada by
AGMV-Marquis Imprimeur Inc.
2700, rue Rachel, est
Montréal, (Québec) H2H 1S7

Words of Wisdom Press
30765 Pacific Coast Hwy., #266
Malibu, California 90265
1-888-746-1593
www.drbillcode.com

Canadian Cataloguing in Publication Data:

William E. Code, MD, FRCPC (Anesthesiology)
Denise Code, MSc (Nutrition), RD
[Who's in Control of your Multiple Sclerosis?]

Who's in Control of your Multiple Sclerosis?
PIECES OF THE MS RECOVERY PUZZLE
Cover Design by: Chameleon Design & Communications
Duncan, British Columbia

PRINTED IN CANADA

What People Are Saying

"I want to congratulate you for daring to pursue a healing path even though that meant straying far from what you learned in medical school. I find that a great many people come to Integrative Medicine because they first realized its potential in their own life. I trust many are finding benefit in applying what you have learned. Certainly your vitamin D chapter makes perfect sense, and I think conventional medicine will rapidly catch up to what you are saying in the coming years."

Larry Willms, MD, Sioux Lookout, Ontario

"Words cannot express our gratitude to you for writing such an excellent book. It has been really helpful."

Cathy Preyra, Ottawa, Ontario

"I loved the book. It gave me confidence and it reinforced that I was doing things right for my health."

Suzi Ness, Alaska

"I just finished reading your book *Who's in Control of Your MS*. I found the book very helpful in providing alternative therapies for MS."

Kelsey Hoffo

"How many books have been written on alternative healing! Now and then one appears which actually offers something new and helpful. *Who's in Control of Your Multiple Sclerosis* is one of those rare, easy-to-read exceptions.

But there is more here than empathy and an encouragement to 'take charge' of one's life. Dr. Code carefully outlines a comprehensive set of tools by which chronic sufferers can help minimize their afflictions and, hopefully, reverse their conditions. *Who's in Control* is packed with coping and healing strategies, such as the chapter on dietary supplements that could serve by itself as a stand-alone primer. This chapter is something even healthy individuals would find helpful, along with the closing section on Dr. Code's 10 Choices for Chronic Illness."

Paul Rothe, Victoria, British Columbia

"I consider Dr. Bill Code my wellness coach. Together with his wife, Denise, Dr. Code has made a significant impact on my overall health and wellness through his book *Who's in Control of Your MS* and his personal recommendations. As a person living with MS for 37 years, the importance of managing a chronic illness effectively cannot be overemphasized. Dr. Code's writings and lectures have provided me with valuable information on how to maximize my wellness through proper diet and informed supplementation. I attribute my good health, including weight control, pain relief and sleep management to Dr. Code's straightforward and well-researched recommendations."

Christopher R. Fortune, M.A.
Graduate Certified Executive Coach,
Victoria, British Columbia

"Your book served as a reminder that there is always more we can do for ourselves to improve our health. My hope is that people not just read your book, but that they put into action the things you suggest."

Wendy Bowen, Physiotherapist,
Duncan, British Columbia

"I'm feeling great. My neurologist actually said I've improved from last year. Thanks for your support, Bill."

Jock MacDougall,
Vancouver, British Columbia

"Have read your book – it is excellent ... Thank you for publishing a book that covers alternative ways to deal with this chronic disease – it is not fun to have."

Carol Foster, Administrative Government Assistant,
Victoria, British Columbia

"I have read your books but when I finished the last book you gave me, when we were at Edgar and Ruby's, I was so overwhelmed by your story I cannot help but write to you. Your thoughts, your pain, the frustration, and how you have worked your way to what you are today is truly an amazing victory.

Years ago when I first heard you had MS, you were in my thoughts very often. I prayed that you might be able to help carry on and use your talents.

Thank God, that has happened with much effort on your part, you didn't give up and I marvel at how energetic you are.

I pray for your future years that you can keep on doing what you are doing now.

Bill and Denise, you will always be in my thoughts and prayers!"

Tina Harder – 85 years old,
Saskatoon, Saskatchewan

"Dr. Code,

You have made a difference in my outlook after my diagnosis of M.S. You have answered so many questions about the condition. I now know which vitamins and minerals to take and how to live my best life.

Thank you for your book, which I have read in detail so I feel more confident about my future."

Diane Needleman, RN, Key West Florida

Acknowledgements

Thanks to my family, my Mom, Alice Code, and, of course, our three kids – now all in their twenties — Laura, Brian and Warren. Also, thanks to proofreader/editor Marion Ferguson. Thank you to Capital Region Chapter MS Society of B.C., MS Canada. Key people with the MS network are Jeanette Hughes, Christopher Fortune, Jan Yuill, Ann Muir, Bonnie Pashak, Brenda Adam-Smith and Paul McNamara. Special thank-you to Terri Smith for her Herculean efforts of organization, graphics, word processing and a major contribution on aromatherapy in the "Senses" chapter.

Preface

My initial plan was to have Dr. Paty write the 'foreword' to our book. I have, instead, included a dedication to him, due to his untimely death in December 2004. He and I developed a collegial relationship due to our similar medical, research and clinical paths. My goal with this book is to return more hope to those of us with MS – and to our families.

I have not attempted to replace my medical colleagues. Our neurologists are absolutely key for diagnosis. Neurologists, in conjunction with general (family) practitioners and selected other specialists use all pharmaceutical choices, to the best of their abilities in MS. Neither have I focused on particular herbal or other alternative medications. As an experienced and formerly academic anesthesiologist, I know too well, the potential negative interactions between these and drugs of today.

Denise and I have aimed to teach about any food or safe food supplement that may be helpful to each of us in our own individual health journey. Knowledge within the book could help anyone with chronic illness or even striving toward optimal health. I would like to twice quote Hippocrates, the father of western medicine as we know it. Firstly, he said, "Let food be your medicine." Secondly was his famous quote we can all strive for: "Firstly, do no harm." My entire medical career has focused on the balancing of "cost versus benefit" ratio, or benefits of an agent, versus its downsides or negative side effects. It is from this consideration that the term "balanced anesthesia" was coined. Similarly, it is where I first used the term, "balanced analgesia", as to the using of several different drugs for the optimal acute or chronic pain relief solution.

Our secondary title, "Pieces of the MS Recovery Puzzle", lends itself to many components of our overall well-being – mind, body and spirit. Not all of the puzzle pieces outlined will work for all of us. Instead, we aim to provide a roadmap of where to begin your personal (MS or otherwise) health journey. In addition, this should produce little or no conflict with current western medicine focused solutions.

It is in the book written by MS neurologists, "Multiple Sclerosis, The Guide To Treatment and Management", that Dr. Murray urges people with MS to take more control of their personal choices. The "will and/or hope" to get well partly comes from within each of us. Only we can walk our personal journey. I believe we have given you food for thought as to the many choices now available.

Dr. Bill Code, MD
March 2005

Dedication To
Dr. Donald Winston Paty
(1936-2004)

I first met Dr. Don Paty in July of 1996. He was just back from his own health crisis of eighteen months. This was lymphoma cancer, treated with a bone marrow transplant. Few things can modify our outlook or "wake us up" more than a brush with our own mortality. I sincerely appreciated his teaching, patience and wisdom on MS. My background in neuroscience research, clinical anesthesiology and pain management sped up my education about MS by him a great deal. Similarly, he treated me as a colleague with MS. Later that fall of 1996, when I personally visited Dr. Ali Rajput, Neuroscience Chief, University of Saskatchewan, I learned Dr. Paty was one of the best MS Neurologists on the planet. This is high praise from an experienced academic neurologist such as Dr. Rajput.

In "Lives Lived", of the Canadian Globe and Mail, February 24, 2005, Dr. John M. Thompson described Don Paty as a, "medical researcher, lover of Mozart, Chinese food and JoAnne Paty". Dr. Paty's father was a medical missionary. Don brought his parents' idealism to the single-minded goal of unraveling the puzzle of multiple sclerosis. He displayed dedication, organizational skills, and ability to identify a problem and deal with it. Following his MD at Emory University, he did his neurology training at Duke. Then, after a research fellowship in Newcastle-Upon-Tyne, England, he joined the Neuroscience Department at the University of Western Ontario, London, Canada. He worked closely with his colleagues to establish a multiple sclerosis research clinic at the London Health Sciences Centre.

In 1980, the University of British Columbia, Canada, recruited him to become head of Neurology there, which he held until 1996. He was honoured numerous times for his research and service by medical associations in Canada, the U.S. and Britain. In June 2004, Dr. Paty was awarded the Canadian Meritorious Service Medal for his pioneering work with his colleagues in the use of MRI for the diagnosis and treatment of MS. He will be sorely missed by both colleagues and patients.

Dr. Bill Code MD
March 2005

"The doctor of the future will give little medicine,
but will interest his patients in the care of the human frame,
in diet and in the cause and prevention of disease."

— *Thomas A. Edison*

"Let food be thy medicine and thy medicine be food."

— *Hippocrates*

Contents

Chapter 1

Beginning The Journey

Where were you at 42? Or, where do you see yourself at 42? At 42, I was at the height of a challenging and hectic career in medicine. I was looking forward to continued success and satisfaction in my work. I was enjoying family life and the community in which I lived. Life was indeed good. I did not expect to have to retire from practicing medicine at 42 years of age. At 42, I was diagnosed with multiple sclerosis and could no longer work.

As a typical workaholic male, I had wrapped my self-esteem into a commitment to helping others. I had seriously neglected the development of my own personal self-worth. All of a sudden, my reason for being, as a breadwinner, was taken away from me. I was reeling from the huge blows to my self-image.

I learned the hard way that what really matters in life are personal relationships – those with your partner, family and close friends. Work relationships are seldom as satisfying; I found that professional support is incredibly rare within medicine. During my first year away from work, only three colleagues contacted me. This lack of support was a great disappointment to me during a time of illness and stress. I went from being chair of the Medical Advisory Committee in our local hospital to being described as unsafe to work in any part of anesthesiology. In an effort to regain my privileges at the hospital, I was forced to get legal assistance from the Canadian Medical Protective Association. The anger and pain over this issue between friends and colleagues became intense. The hospital's Medical Advisory Committee was split on the issue; it seemed that the surgical specialists sided with the remaining anesthetists in wanting to prevent my return to medicine. Meanwhile, most family practitioners and other medical specialists could see my side of the situation.

Thus began my own personal journey in dealing with illness and striving towards health. After eight months of effort in medical retraining and after regaining my hospital privileges, I worked on Fridays for only three weeks before noticing that I felt worse. It had all been in vain.

I finally realized that until I could let go of the anger and "poor me" complex, I could not move on. I was the only variable that could be changed in this scenario. It took me more than a year to appreciate that I was the only one who could have a significant impact on my chronic illness of multiple sclerosis. After some time, I began to benefit from empowering myself to make a difference for *me*. This book is intended to outline for the reader some of the steps in my journey – a journey that has been made possible by my earlier understanding of medicine. Every step in this journey has been greatly assisted by my wife and co-author, Denise. I would like to tell you how I arrived at this time of crisis in 1996 and how I emerged, making new dreams from shattered ones.

I am the fifth of seven children and was raised on a small mixed farm in Saskatchewan. I left this small community to study medicine at the University of Saskatchewan in Saskatoon. Following this, I interned at St. Paul's Hospital in Saskatoon and completed an additional six months of anesthesia training. This was in preparation for a rural general practice with two colleagues in Hudson Bay, Saskatchewan. In my four years there, I diagnosed three people with multiple sclerosis and missed diagnosing at least one other.

In 1983, Denise and I decided to move to Calgary where I would do a specialty in anesthesiology and intensive care. We moved with our two young sons, Warren & Brian, and in early 1984 we were delighted at the birth of our daughter, Laura. During the five years in Calgary, I spent two years doing brain research. This involved lab work in the Department of Pharmacology and Anesthesiology as to how anesthetics worked on the brain, and it meant that my career was taking more of an academic turn. It was also at that time that I was fortunate to complete my board exams in both Canada and the United States.

Despite offers for further training at Stanford University in California and a clinical research position at M.D. Anderson Hospital in Houston, we decided to return to Saskatoon, where I joined the Faculty of Medicine. This started a delightful, and yet very hectic four years. I became the Research Director in the Department of Anesthesiology and within a year, had become the Residency Program Director as well. I continued to do research on the brain and was successful, along with several other colleagues, in attaining $1 million research grant from the Heart and Stroke Foundation. However, at this same time, most of my health markers were deteriorating. My cholesterol continued to climb; my blood pressure was elevated and my migraine headaches were so frequent I would use a large bottle of extra strength acetaminophen every month.

In 1990, in Duncan, on Vancouver Island on the West Coast, I visited a colleague that I had trained with in Calgary. He invited me to join him in clinical practice. In the spring of 1992, Denise and I decided to do just that. Prior to leaving Saskatoon, I was particularly impacted by the movie, "Regarding Henry", starring Harrison Ford. The message it conveyed to me was that, despite the huge problem Henry had with his health, his life actually improved when he stepped out of his hectic legal practice in New York. This was the first time I was able to admit to Denise that I was a workaholic.

A move at this time was a particular challenge for our oldest son, Warren, who was about to start high school. Even so, he was extremely generous and understanding. He said that we would make the right decision. I still appreciate his sensitivity and wisdom in accepting such a great change in our lives. By moving to the West Coast, I was, of course, leaving behind clinical research and clinical teaching. This meant my workload was decidedly less but permitted much more time to spend with my family. All of my stress-related health markers improved in that first-year. In fact, the Financial Post Fortune 500 magazine had a feature article on me, calling me the "Quintessential Baby Boomer". I was typical of the individual leaving his very hectic life in the city for a more relaxed laid-back life in a smaller center. A framed picture of the article remains in our home today.

Like many workaholics, one is only a "recovering workaholic", because one is never completely healed. Within a year of moving to Vancouver Island, I started to see people for chronic and acute pain problems. This was almost always for one to three hours at the end of the operating room day. Chronic and acute pain issues are both primarily concerned with the function of the nervous system. Two of my earliest patients had multiple sclerosis. One was helped with epidural injections that enabled her to sit down without extreme discomfort. The other one had such severe muscle spasms that he had an infusion pump placed in his abdomen to deliver a drug, baclofen, continuously into his cerebrospinal fluid. At least once a month, I was responsible for refilling the pump with baclofen and supervising its delivery over 24 hours.

My ongoing interest in acute pain issues had resulted in my publishing a number of research articles and an editorial in the Canadian Journal of Anesthesiology. My editorial was titled "Balanced Analgesia". My involvement with chronic pain, primarily while in private practice, resulted in my being invited to Australia in April 1996. I was one of the few Canadians asked to speak at the World Congress of Anesthesiology being held in Sydney. My topic was "how to treat pain without the use of opiates" (narcotics). It was very exciting to be speaking to some 2500 people, with pictures of myself across the front of the stage, leaving me nowhere to hide!

After returning home from the Congress of Anesthesiology, I started to notice it was getting harder and harder to recover from my on-call nights. I was still cycling the six kilometers to work, but my right foot would frequently slip off the pedal and I would nearly fall. By early July, I chose to drive to and from work as a safer option. By then it was hard to recover from any day's work. I found it difficult to get up in the mornings and I remained groggy, despite going to bed at 9 or 10 o'clock at night. If it had been a busy call-night in anesthesia and I was working most of a 24-hour period, even after an entire day of rest, I did not feel recovered. In fact, I still didn't feel recovered by the time it was my turn to go back on-call again three days later.

I noticed other changes. My right foot would slap at times when I walked, especially if I was tired. In addition, I was finding it more difficult to see my chronic pain clients for the usual two to three hours at the end of the operating room day. I had noticed a peculiar problem – the long, hollow needles I used for epidural injections seemed to be getting quite dull. I contacted the company's representative and she was very quick to send out two new boxes of needles. However they were no better and it puzzled me. Finally, in early July, I made an appointment for a checkup with my family doctor. She examined me and suggested I see a neurologist. I was seen soon thereafter by a University of British Columbia neurologist. He found many more signs and symptoms: significant hyperreflexia (over-reactive reflexes) on my right side, lateral gaze nystagmus, right-sided weakness, a positive Romberg's test, poor ability to track on the finger to nose test, and an inability to walk with one foot directly in front of the other. He also noted that I had a much reduced sensation on my right side and that I was up three to four times a night to empty my bladder. By the end of the interview, he had booked me for an MRI. When he reviewed me two weeks later, he recommended I take six months off work because he believed I had multiple sclerosis.

I was devastated. So was my family. Denise and our eldest son, Warren, who were with me at the time of my Vancouver neurologist appointment, tried to support me. I said to Denise, "I feel like I am worth more dead than alive." I saw myself continuing to slide straight down the slope of diminished strength, balance and energy. I anticipated progressive incapacity, even incontinence, needing to leave home for hospital, then an institution and early death. My neurologist believed that progressive multiple sclerosis was more probable, because my situation had worsened continuously over the last four months.

By the time I left work on August 23rd, 1996, I was having someone drive me to work. I stumbled around the operating room and seriously discussed with my coworkers the pros and cons of a three-wheel or four-wheel scooter for myself. I was unable to empty a syringe with my right hand, and both of my hands were so numb, that procedures such as starting epidurals or intravenous needles were done solely on a visual basis. My diagnosis and major right-sided weakness explained one of my summer mysteries. I remembered that I had complained to the needle sales representative that their product seemed extraordinarily dull. The replacement needles had been no better. By the time I was diagnosed by the neurologist, the "penny had dropped". I realized that the epidural needles had been fine, but that the strength in my right hand had disappeared so gradually and insidiously, that I had not realized that my hands were the problem.

For the next nine months, I continued to worsen. My depth of field vision (distance perception) was terrible. Even as a car passenger, I drove the driver to distraction and frustration. I worried that almost anyone would hit us at an intersection, or at a streetlight. I know now that eighty percent of multiple sclerosis patients are diagnosed with changes in their vision. Even though my case was not so severe, I now have a much better understanding of their fear and frustration.

Sleep: there was never enough. Even after 12 to 13 hours of rest, I would still feel like my arms and legs were nailed down to the bed. I often took an afternoon nap for one or two hours. One afternoon, as I awoke from my nap, I saw a hand in bed beside me. I had no concept of where this hand had come from. It was my hand. My whole sense of proprioception (awareness of where our limbs are) was almost gone. In fewer than six months, I'd gone from being able to play pretty fair ping-pong or tennis to having terrible eye-hand coordination.

Worse still, I was so irritable that, after lunch, my family would often specifically request that I have a nap. My uncontrollable irritability put tremendous stress on the relationships between my closest family members and myself. The chronic fatigue, coupled with my anger toward everything, especially myself, started to alienate my teenage sons, Brian and Warren. They became very reluctant to help me, no matter how small the request might be. My temper fuse was so short that they came to see my constant blowups as inevitable. My senses of vision, hearing and even smell were so incredibly oversensitive, that any small incident would trigger my anger. The term "naked nerve endings" was a common description, and in reality, I guess it was correct!

I distinctly remember the Christmas season of 1996. Our immediate family decided to drive the 1200 kilometers to Regina, Saskatchewan. This would enable Denise and I to see each of our siblings, and allow our kids to visit their cousins in both Regina and Calgary. To start, we took the ferry from Vancouver Island to Vancouver, British Columbia. It was dark by the time we docked at Tsawwassen terminal on the mainland side. Denise was driving and I was navigating (or at least trying to). We were supposed to meet and pickup our oldest son, Warren, who had just completed his first term at the University of British Columbia in Vancouver. Over the next 30 minutes, I proceeded to get Denise and our other two children hopelessly lost. Finally our son Brian navigated. He was fed up with the recurrent bickering back and forth between Denise and myself. I realized that there were more problems now than I had anticipated happening within my brain. My complete inability to navigate with the map both frustrated and frightened me; I had lost a significant skill, with which I had once excelled since my time as a Boy Scout. This was my first significant encounter with the cognitive component of multiple sclerosis. Up to sixty percent of people with multiple sclerosis have significant cognitive problems. These include issues with problem solving, reading maps, short-term memory, and multitasking, as well as the development of what may be referred to as "brain fog".

With Brian at the wheel, we found Warren about ten minutes later, but our trip did not improve. I was a major hassle and frustration to all my fellow travelers. I couldn't tolerate the flashing car lights, any kind of music jangled my ears and I was soon very irritable, as even modest bumps in the road made sleep impossible for me. The bumps would trigger shooting electrical pain, with or without muscle spasms, into one or both legs. Seventy percent of people with multiple sclerosis suffer from one or both of these symptoms badly enough to seek medication or treatment. Unfortunately this nerve irritability pain (neuropathic pain) is notoriously hard to treat. By the time we reached Regina, my family was almost ready to give me away. My multiple sclerosis had turned a happy trip into a near nightmare.

When I returned to my neurologist in the new year, it had been five months since my diagnosis and I was no better. In reality, I was worse than when I left work. My neurologist answered my question, "What do I do next?" with "You need to take another six months off." This statement made me realize two truths; No. 1: Western medicine has very little to offer chronic illness and No. 2: if I was going to have any control over my recovery, then I would have to learn all I could about my own illness.

I became aware of how fast and furious I had been running in my practice of medicine. It took months before I appreciated this little known fact. Most of my medical colleagues routinely run on a similar treadmill, resulting in great costs to themselves, their families and eventually their own health. I've been told that the average lifespan of a physician in North America is 56 years; without a doubt, I know very few old anesthesiologists.

In February 1997, my dad, was diagnosed with lymphoma at the age of 79. At that time, I had already returned to my role as tenor in a local choir. My seatmate in the choir, a pathologist, remarked to me that my father's lymphoma was one of the nastiest and most aggressive cases that he had ever seen. This was another major blow. My dad and I had always been extremely close. I decided not to discuss this grim prognosis with him. Instead, we six siblings (after losing a brother to AIDS in 1994) pulled together to support our parents. After many unsuccessful radiation treatments, my father gave chemotherapy a try. In addition to many hazardous side effects, this too, proved ineffective. Several of us, including me, were starting to look outside traditional Western medicine in reaction to Dad's losing battle with cancer. However, we were unsuccessful. He passed away at home in mid-September of that year. For me it had seemed as though he had hung on until I had received back my hospital privileges, which came through two days before he died. This had been a goal of mine that had required several months of struggle to achieve, and he knew how important it was to me.

Following a week's refresher training in Victoria, I was booked for three successive Fridays to work in our local operating room, but by the third Friday, I was much worse again. I had to recognize that something in the operating room milieu was having a negative impact on my health. Had I proved myself wrong regarding anesthesia and its "non worsening" of MS symptoms? Absolutely. This was another bitter pill to swallow. Maybe, just maybe, I had to look beyond the regular boundaries of accepted medical practice for relief of my own progressive multiple sclerosis.

By now it was the latter part of 1997. I had learned of an upcoming conference in Vancouver about complementary and alternative methods to either slow down or assist my tolerance of MS symptoms. I attended, and the conference was a whole new experience. I was placed together with a large number of people who had multiple sclerosis at all stages and ages. I felt very lucky to still be able to walk, albeit with a limp. More importantly, I realized that many others were seeking new options in their own journey with this chronic illness.

The conference proved to be my introduction to the Paleolithic Diet or Stone Age Diet. I went on this Stone Age Diet. I stayed on it for almost a month and then, not seeing any changes, I gave it up. However, it did make a huge impact on me insofar as convincing me of the possibility that I might be able to control my MS. Denise and I started to look at diet changes we could implement or what particular nutritional supplements might make a difference in my multiple sclerosis.

This ongoing work is the reason for writing this book. We share with you, the reader, choices that may have a significant impact on your journey to health or that of a loved one. None of these recommendations are risky or harmful. Nor are they intended to replace your neurologist or family physician. Rather, these choices can complement traditional medical therapies. That is, these choices can be implemented along with any treatment prescribed by your doctor. Our only request is that you keep an open mind and keep your own healthcare practitioner in the loop. Once again, I must emphasize that you should know more about your chronic illness than does your family doctor. You are empowering yourself if you proceed on this journey.

Chapter 2

How We Can Impact
Our Health Journey?

Multiple sclerosis, in its simplest form, is believed to be an autoimmune disease. In short, some of the body's own white blood cells are attacking the myelin (insulation lining) of the nerve cells in the brain and spinal cord (CNS). Meanwhile, the nerves, muscle and skin outside the CNS are normal and are not under attack. Over time, the entire lining of the myelin sheath may be removed and nerves are left without insulation. This permits incorrect messaging to occur or so-called short-circuiting. Eventually, many of these naked nerves or axons will die.

Whenever injury occurs in our bodies, the body responds with an attempt to heal itself using a process of inflammation, which includes swelling, redness, heat and pain or loss of function. This same process is triggered whether it occurs in an ankle sprain or whether it results from our own white blood cells attacking tissue in the brain and spinal cord. The initial problems with an attack of MS are usually partly or largely due to the swelling component. This is why corticosteroids work, because hopefully, they shorten the attack. However, we also realize that they do not benefit the illness of MS in the long term. This is an important distinction as it may help the individual to decide whether or not to use corticosteroids. Of course corticosteroids come with certain side effects such as early cataracts, osteoporosis, peptic ulcers, mood changes and even occasionally the loss of a hip joint (avascular necrosis). The side effects are very important considerations in our cost-benefit decision, as in other parts of health and medicine. When the body completes the inflammation process in its efforts to heal, we are left with the scar or sclerosis. A series of several scars in the CNS is described by the term *multiple sclerosis.* The scars show as white spots or patches on an image produced by magnetic resonance imaging (MRI).

How then can we as individuals control our MS? From the above description of the white blood cells attacking our nerves, inflammation and eventual scarring, there are several steps where we may be able to influence things:

1. Prevent what triggers the change in our white blood cell group.
2. Reduce the ability of this white blood cell group to gain access to the CNS (i.e. across the blood brain barrier).
3. Reduce the inflammation and free radicals that damage the initial cells and also the surrounding cells.
4. Alter our diet to provide building blocks so that injured cells in the CNS can be repaired or new healthy replacement cells can be generated.

Today, none of these can be accomplished completely or 100 percent. Hence, we must aim for partial improvement, with as few negative side effects as possible. If we can achieve several 10 to 15 percent pieces of the puzzle, then we can have an impact or start to control our illness. We are not talking about a cure. We are talking about making a difference to ourselves. Recognize that, over a period of 7 to 8 years, every single cell of our seventy trillion cells is replaced by a new cell.

It has recently been discovered that healing can occur in the brain and spinal cord; this has only been accepted in the last decade. One concession that multiple sclerosis does offer its victims is time. What we are suggesting is that it is up to the individual to empower him- or herself to make a difference in his or her own health. Thus, even if we are only partly successful, we will still greatly enhance our outlook and potentially, our outcome as well.

The remainder of this chapter will outline some of the steps that seem reasonable and have worked for others and me. None of the steps are harmful to anyone and so there is little to lose in trying them. The first principle learned in medical school is Hippocrates' statement, "Primum nom nocere" — "do no harm". Every time we use a drug in anesthesiology, it is always with the concept of the risk-benefit ratio in mind. We follow that dictum in our everyday life and this book aims to do this as well.

One of the choices we recommend is a regular intake of omega-3 fatty acids. Our personal favorite is brown flax, finely ground and DHA from fish oil or krill oil. There are a number of reasons for this. Firstly, by increasing our omega-3 intake we are counterbalancing the significant amount of inflammation from excess omega-6 fatty acids. Most of us in North America take in 12 to 18 times as many omega-6 fatty acids as omega-3 fatty acids. For this reason we do not recommend or advocate oil supplementation as being limited to gamma linolenic acid (GLA), which is usually obtained from evening primrose oil. Omega-3 fatty acids are also the most effective building blocks in our brain and spinal cord (CNS). Our brain is almost 60 percent fat and the omega-3 fatty acids are the dominant component of this fat. One chapter will deal with omega-3 fatty acids, saturated fats and trans fats in considerable detail.

Vitamin D, the sunshine vitamin, has a stunning story to reveal to us. We will show vitamin D to be the great sleeper vitamin. You will learn the regions where multiple sclerosis is dominant in Australia, relative to the equator. Researchers were able to follow this premise and relate it to the amount of ultraviolet light received in different regions of Australia. In addition, we will discuss the relative advantages of living near an ocean coast and of eating plenty of cold-water fish. Finally, you will learn the minimum and the maximum amount of vitamin D that you can safely take. This can now be readily measured by your health care practitioner. You'll discover why this supplement is (fortunately) inexpensive. Side benefits will be such things as helping reduce blood pressure, slow osteoporosis and minimize some cancers including bowel, breast and prostate. We now know that if you give an infant 1000 international units of vitamin D per day they will have markedly less risk of developing multiple sclerosis, rheumatoid arthritis, childhood cancers and even juvenile onset diabetes mellitus.

In a later chapter, we will both confess and explain why we no longer simply eat a well-balanced diet and why we should all take a multivitamin/mineral supplement as the minimum of any dietary intake. We will describe how this is a very useful adjunct to both Canada's food guide and the U.S. food pyramid. Our discussion will help you understand why it is not wise to just guess which vitamins and minerals we should supplement. An example of this would be vitamin E, which can be supplemented at 400 units but at 800 units usually does more harm than good. Key features within that multivitamin are folic acid, vitamin B12 and vitamin B6. Anyone with multiple sclerosis should ensure that they have an adequate intake of these key vitamins; this not only reduces the risk of developing multiple sclerosis but also reduces neural tube defects (spina bifida), spontaneous abortions or miscarriages and the significant component of heart disease, homocysteine. Finally, we will introduce the concept of antioxidants. We will outline where one can look for these within whole foods.

Calcium and magnesium are also discussed. This is because anyone with reduced activity and exercise is at very high risk of osteoporosis. Certainly MS people fit into this group - even more so if corticosteroids are part of their treatment regimen. Calcium and magnesium are also critically important for the ideal function of all cells including nerve cells. Magnesium is often used for irritable heart cells, particularly the pacemaker types of cells. Similarly, it has a significant role in the improvement of nerve cell irritability in the brain and spinal cord. In fact, it is still used today to avoid seizures in the final stage of toxemia in pregnancy. This discussion of calcium and magnesium will tie in with the Vitamin D chapter, as you learn how it is possible to take much less expensive calcium because of the supplementation of the vitamin D.

Why would anybody apply or swallow emu oil? The reasons for this will be outlined, including all the current research. Also included, will be the concept that emu oil is recognized as an anti-inflammatory drug in Australia. Some people will apply emu oil or a pain mixture containing emu oil to reduce both pain and muscle spasms. A number of other natural product approaches will be discussed. These include things like ginkgo biloba, ginseng and other potential energy tonics. Whenever these items are used, we want everyone to consider the risk-benefit ratio. If, after this consideration, it seems a reasonable way to proceed, then go for it!

We recommend that you avoid or minimize foods to which you know you are, or may be, sensitive. This discussion will include the anthropological approach in the Paleolithic or Stone Age diet, and some interesting genetic issues regarding MS; for example, the predisposition to MS of people who originate from Northern Europe. Is there any logical basis to the "eat right for your blood type" theory? The short answer is yes. We will suggest why Canada actually has the highest incidence of inflammatory bowel disease in the world. How does this and the leaky gut syndrome potentially link with multiple sclerosis, or does it? Finally, why do I avoid modern wheat or pasta as do many Central Europeans? In fact, an increasing number of West coasters in North America do so as well. It is here that you will find a commentary on grains that probably you have never heard of before, such as spelt, kamut, amaranth and other ancient, yet now, new foods.

Exercise — why bother, or better yet, why work with an enlightened physio or personal trainer? We will describe how it is often possible to retrain both our balance as well as our backup motor nerve pathways. Fortunately, the Master Designer (he or she) gave us five times as many motor nerve pathways as we typically use in a lifetime. Many of our proprioceptive or position senses are in reality miniature motor nerve pathways. By focusing and concentrating in front of a mirror, we can potentially regain or improve our balance and walking. A number of significant people have contributed to this exciting chapter and its concepts. Certainly Feldenkrais is the forerunner responsible for many of these practical and useful techniques. Similarly, Meir Schneider, Montell Williams and our Canadian, Eva Marsh, have given us techniques and stories about how practical and achievable this is. These methods have worked for me, a skeptical physician, and we have seen them work for others as well. Mind, body and spirit are powerful tools to help all of us along the way.

Immune system optimizers and modulators, including Vitamin D, flax, multivitamin/minerals and glutathione are also discussed in this book. Glutathione is a tripeptide (a protein with three amino acids) that must be made inside every cell of the body, including our brain cells and white blood cells. It is now recognized that glutathione is the key and master antioxidant within our body. Until recently, we have never had a way to boost or increase the glutathione inside the cells safely, with minimal or no side effects. Now, a whey protein isolate has been found that can refurbish the glutathione inside these white blood cells. In addition, this whey protein isolate is rarely a cause of allergic reaction.

Concepts of energy production and fatigue problems will be reviewed in detail. Taking an amount of this whey protein isolate every day has been a large piece of the puzzle for my energy recovery, lost because of my MS. While I must insist that this is not a magic bullet (there are no magic bullets in medicine or nutrition), I do believe that this discovery of the building blocks of glutathione is the most significant step forward in our health care since penicillin was discovered. Further details will be discussed as to why the glutathione already in our diet is not helpful in producing glutathione inside the cells. There will also be discussion about how the drug N-acetyl cysteine (NAC) is able to only temporarily raise the glutathione in most body cells but is unable to cross the blood brain barrier, a significant limitation to those of us with multiple sclerosis or those with other brain troubles related to oxidative stress.

"Detoxification" is an oft used and oft misquoted term, and this subject alone warrants a chapter. To an anesthesiologist, detoxification means the removal of drugs and drug byproducts from a cell and from the body. This applies in particular to drugs acting on the brain and spinal cord. It also applies to toxic components from our environment. These would include things like herbicides, pesticides, heavy metals, and large numbers of petrochemical or cleaning agents. The key substance in our body for removing almost every drug used in medicine or anesthesiology is glutathione. Now that we know how to optimize or raise the glutathione in every cell, we are now able to do an ongoing, safe and continuous detoxification. This will only assist those of us who have an illness that is partly aggravated due to sensitivity to substances which injure or affect brain cells.

The final chapter will discuss in further detail the journey experienced by the authors with their experience as "MS person" and "MS caregiver" respectively. Both Denise and I indeed feel fortunate that we had a great deal of knowledge and wisdom before the onset of multiple sclerosis. Our marriage of 29 years, has been enlightened and fuelled by a Master's Degree in Nutrition on one side, plus extensive work in brain and stroke research, pharmacology and physiology, on the other side. The synergy of the above when combined with the much-improved communication in our world today, has made this book possible and we hope you find it worthwhile. You (or someone you care about) may be on a personal journey with multiple sclerosis or some other chronic illness. Our goal is to make this book a source of practical and usable health information, supplemented by updates at our web site, **www.emu.ca**.

Chapter 3

MS Society, Networks and Impact on Wellness

As I previously mentioned how I became part of our local MS Society, I will now outline why and how important this can be. I believe we underestimate how the importance of our interaction with other human beings is. Indeed, our MS illness often diminishes our relationships within our workplace and even in our own community. My busy medical practice, including operating room anesthesiology, acute pain rounds and chronic pain outpatients, dramatically reduced my interpersonal contacts outside of work.

This was obvious and necessary due to the tremendous fatigue I was experiencing. It also put a strain on my interaction with medical colleagues, as they no longer knew how to interact with me. Now, eight years later, I can see how huge an impact this had on my own recovery. I, too, need relationships and personal interaction to operate fully as a human being. Maybe part of this is being the fifth of seven children. Perhaps it developed through my enjoyment of sixty-five classmates in medical school and 15-20 colleagues during internship and anesthesia residency.

This social gap was gradually filled by my involvement with the local MS Society support group, MS Society Board participation and even national and some international participation.

Most of this began due to the effort and energy expended on me by Helen Catherall, an occupational therapist employed part-time by the Vancouver Island MS Society, who helped me regain my social networks. She met me at a local restaurant for coffee and spent time with me and my well-being. She started with simple physical and emotional issues. She suggested our family meet with the MS Chapter Social Worker to establish a baseline of how each of us was coping with my MS diagnosis and changes. She also addressed my difficulties with the disability pension plan application and refusals. She diplomatically outlined why an automobile handicapped parking sign or sticker could save my meager energy supply. Finally, she described the function of the local MS Society and Board and how I could be helpful to them. The latter was partly due to my research and grantsmanship experience in brain and stroke research on two university campuses. This helped my self-esteem, in demonstrating that I was still valuable to my community.

Soon after, I began to come out of my self-imposed isolation and withdrawal, I began to move on from "poor me" or "no value me" to becoming a team player again in the game of life. For example, the handicap parking sticker was useful, both for parking and for me recognizing that I was part of a "challenged" or "special needs" group. It was also a part of my "coming out" or admitting to others that I had a chronic illness. This is a tough step for many of us. I have met people who have "closeted" their MS for five to twenty years. Certainly, denial is a useful defense mechanism but even more important is the next step of personal interaction, cooperative education, support and, yes, the power of new friendships.

I still remember the relief of parking near the door of the grocery store. Yes, I could have a little extra energy to push the grocery cart! I had already learned that a grocery cart was an "invisible" walking aid, acceptable to others and myself. My daughter, Laura, was initially hesitant to ride with me and park in a handicap-parking stall. She either did not see me as handicapped or, accept me as such. In time, this hesitance eased. I learned even big changes start with small steps.

Soon after meeting Helen, I went to my first local MS support group meeting. This was pretty traumatic. Two thirds of the regular group were using canes, walkers or wheel-chairs. I also saw a man I had sung tenor with in choir for three years. He, too, had just been diagnosed with MS. One of the more outspoken members of the group approached me boldly and insisted I should sign-up to work at the local bingo hall to help support the group through gaming. She stated I should get at it right away, as I was still walking. I have always been poor at saying no and this was no exception. Thankfully, my Mom later offered to fill this time slot in the smoke-filled Bingo hall. I sometimes forget the great support I have received. Unfortunately, the meeting of a high propor-tion of people who were walking-challenged further skewed my long-term outlook and hope. To this point, I mostly had seen MS compromised individuals in a hospital setting and see-ing them in a community setting did nothing to raise my spirits.

Helen's visit also led to my introduction with Paul McNamara, the Executive Director of the Victoria-based MS Society Chapter. He was fairly new in his role there and was looking for Society Board members to fulfill particular needs. We hit it off well and he introduced me to a large set of use-ful and supportive resources. Helen and Paul soon had me enrolled in a 12-member, newly diagnosed group. This was led by Bonnie Pashak, a talented and passionate social work-er of the MS Society. Within two months, I was a new Board member representing my area of Duncan and fulfilling the role of novelty specialist physician with a neuroscience research background and his own personal MS.

Our newly diagnosed group, led by Bonnie gelled quickly into friendships, trust and mutual support. We were all hungry for stories similar to our own so that we could realize we were "not the only one" with this peculiar fate. The group was two-thirds women and one-third men –repre-sentative of the population of MS is in Canada. We shared the "but you look so well" which we had all heard so frequently, and we laughed at it. We often cried over other issues of emotional pain, work trials and tribulations. I suspect that it was this emotional roller coaster which Bonnie, our group co-ordinator, guided so patiently, that bonded us together so quickly. In fact, we continued to meet for nearly two years, and some of us are still close friends seven years later. Only now, do I fully appreciate the significance of these contacts. Interaction of like-minded or similarly challenged people makes for more powerful individuals and a unique team approach. Yes, laughter is still the best medicine. I believe most of us started our recovery and our renewed belief in ourselves in this group. Certainly, I did.

This group, the newly-diagnosed, or newly-accepting of a diagnosis of MS, also helped our primary and secondary care-givers in a positive fashion. Spouses or partners were encouraged to come and one of the eight meetings was focused on the caregivers (see Chapter 5 – Caregivers At Home And In The Community). Some of the great weight was taken off their shoulders by their participation. In summary, my recommendation is that all of us diagnosed with MS should participate in a newly-diagnosed / newly-accepting the diagnosis, group. I have added the "newly accepting" or this "coming out" about your MS as one step or stage in your healing process. In my experience, some of us take years to get to this stage. Perhaps it is like the four stages of grieving about death – anger, denial, grief, acceptance. In no uncertain terms, chronic illness is a major turning point in your life. Until we accept and recognize such a change, we cannot fully react, respond or completely "heal" the problem. We are not an illness, but our illness is a component of who we are and how we embrace life thereafter. If we do not win this battle of wills, then our illness can and often does take over, and get the upper hand.

A concurrent event in my journey was becoming a board member in the MS Society chapter based in Victoria. My interaction with this group also became a valuable experience in my personal journey toward wellness. The Board represented some 1300 folks with MS, of a total population of 700,000 people, on Vancouver Island, B.C., Canada. It is one of the most complete physically and emotionally supportive and rehabilitative options in North America. This got my attention, big time. After sliding downhill steadily for thirteen months, I felt I needed an option for family respite, in case the rapid slide continued. Victoria had a 100-110 MS client caseload of frequent and regular visits to the MS centre. The benefits derived, were dramatic and enabled many to stay in their own home and out of institutional care. I admit I wanted to become a part of this group rather run the risk of burdening my family with my total care or face the possibility of being institutionalized. My long-term prognosis looked dismal in late 1997. The rapid advance of my progressive multiple sclerosis was unrelenting. I have a personal habit of wanting to have all my bases covered. I felt that as an active member, I had a good chance of slipping into this long-established core group. Each year, one or two of our members with MS would need to retire from the group due to the worsening of their MS. I did not know when my own number would come up. I had no idea, or long-term hope, of being as recovered as I am now in early 2005!

As a Chapter member in the autumn of 1998, I was asked to attend the International Symposium of Multiple Sclerosis in Cleveland, Ohio, USA. I was excited at the prospect, believing I would discover the latest and greatest options for treatment and rehabilitation of MS. Three weeks prior to this I tried riding a recumbent bicycle previously ridden across Canada by Pierre Doré. After only ten feet, I stopped, fell over and badly smashed my right ankle. This occurred in a back alley on Davy Street in downtown Vancouver. My friends helped me into a van and drove me to nearby St. Paul's Hospital. However, I should have tied my feet together with my shoelaces, as I had learned in Boy Scout First Aid. Once placed on the floor of the van, my right foot plunked over at a right angle to my body, because no bony or tissue support remained! I was fortunate to see a "Top Gun" orthopedic surgeon, Dr. Simon Horlick, who explained I needed two pieces of steel and 5-6 months, of non-weight-bearing time (i.e. wheelchair). Membership in the medical profession does have its privileges; Dr. Horlick asked me if I had any requests in my 28-36 hours wait for an emergency surgery slot. I asked to see an anesthesiologist from the Acute Pain service. My "wish" was granted and he set me up with a push button pump for morphine (PCA or Patient Controlled Analgesic) and a twice-daily dose of oral naproxen, 500 mgs. The two in combination are quite good for bone and soft tissue injury pain control. Just when I thought I was on cloud nine (morphine has been nicknamed "nectar of the gods") I had a rude awakening. The combination of being bed-ridden, on a tricyclic antidepressant, and now morphine, plus my MS, meant I could not empty my bladder. This necessitated urinary catheterization by a young, embarrassed nurse. I had the catheter for several days, almost right up until the time I was discharged from hospital.

My surgery took place some 30 hours after admission – not bad by Canadian standards. I was fitted with an ankle brace and told to stay off my feet. Three weeks later I was Cleveland-bound, wheelchair and all.

My flight from Vancouver to Toronto was relatively uneventful. I was loaded on board the airplane with a mobile board-chair device and had an aisle seat. The flight attendant only hit my cast boot once with the drink and food trolley! It is so great when people learn quickly.

The next issue was transferring from one terminal to another, which included a bus ride, en route to my Toronto-Cleveland airplane. This required the entire two and a half hour stop over. No problem, but it was now seven hours since I had been to a washroom to empty my bladder. Mercifully, both the flight and the Cleveland transport to my hotel were short. The bladder spasms were major and very frequent by then. It sounds like birth labour pains, doesn't it?! I checked in at the desk and made it to my room to go to the washroom, which was a considerable relief. There were more bladder spasms and then relative comfort. For the next three weeks, frequent voids and bladder spasms persisted.

The MS symposium conference was amazing. I felt tickled pink and grateful to my MS Society Board of Directors for sending me as their representative. There were long presentations about MRI changes or non-changes relative to the "Big Three Drugs" – Interferon – 1a, 1b, and Glatimer Acetate. The speakers restated that it was still very difficult, if possible at all, to correlate clinical findings in an MS patient with MRI findings. This is perhaps, where the individual's spirit, doggedness or "control" of their own destiny, steps in. In my eight and a half years with MS, and my meeting of hundreds of MS people, this gap between clinical MRI and clinical status, seems to persist.

At the MS symposium, coffee time or break time was a whole new issue for me. There were two wheelchairs and three scooters among some 400 participants. I have never been so invisible in my life! The experience changed my wheelchair perspective, for life. Nancy Holland, one of the major players in the United States' MS Society, was helpful and instantly recognized my frustration. In addition, she made available two of the pending booklets on Symptom Management of MS complications. These included bladder issues, pain issues and fatigue. They are a very useful algorithm or decision tree pattern for clinicians caring for MS patients. Those of us with MS should access these booklets from our local MS Society for our own knowledge and to share with our primary care physicians. Some neurologists will also benefit, as MS is sometimes a minor portion of their practice.

Information and knowledge are the kingpins to acquire if we are to optimally control our own destiny. This is especially key for those of us living in one of two "hinterlands". This includes rural and also, dense, urban living. Ready access to a MS clinic will minimize this need, but access is not routinely available to many of us with MS. I realize a purist (e.g. MS neurologist) would like to have this information for only confirmed MS cases. However, after my own four years of Family Practice, where pre-diagnosis or pre-disease assessment is common, we need to broaden our scope. I understand the average time to MS diagnosis is still six to seven years. These "waiting to be diagnosed" folks still deserve some symptom management, particularly with non-harmful or non-addicting therapeutic choices. This potential vacuum turns some people outside regular channels, to seek more information, knowledge and even solutions. Our hope is that this book can bridge the gap or at least temporize some of these issues. Certainly the waiting time and the frustration due to the lack of solutions, make these individuals vulnerable to the many friends and neighbours with anecdotes galore. It may be these very different paths that stir the pot of frustration and mistrust between divergent groups. Knowledge, facts, and "do no harm" solutions can help resolve this disparity.

Back to the conference, and time for me to get off my soapbox. The next important consideration is the network of people I met, which included a gathering of Canadian MS Society representatives. We watched an excellent video which taught youngsters what MS in their parent, might look like. For example, mittens simulated loss of touch and double vision eyeglasses simulated vision problems encountered in MS. Of course, we all enjoyed an evening tour of the "Rock 'n Roll" museum. Most of us could relate to the origins of Chubby Checker and Elvis Presley. My report of the Conference to the Board spoke highly of the value of the networking, the forming of relationships and the knowledge gleaned from the meeting. If this sort of activity interests you, get active in your MS Society!

One of the long term goals of our Victoria, Canada-based MS Society, has been easier accessibility to an MS Clinic with MS neurologists and a multi-disciplinary team.

Through the efforts of our MS Society Board in Victoria, the MS Clinic at UBC (University of British Columbia, Vancouver, B.C.), Dr. Joel Oger, and the MS – BC Division, of MS Canada, this easier accessibility came to fruition. The clinic experienced growing pains, but all in all, our efforts improved the plight of diagnosed MS people considerably. This usually eliminated the two-hour ferry ride, each way to and from Vancouver, and the long, long day for a group of very low energy people and their caregivers.

But appointment time and space were almost immediately at a premium. The MS Nurse was pulled in too many directions at once. Resolution was achieved when space was obtained by MS neurologist, Dr. Hrebicek, at the nearby Royal Jubilee Hospital in Victoria. The MS neurologist and MS Nurse moved to the hospital scenario, closer to their pattern of practice and to that of most Canadian MS Clinics. The two-year trial of a solely community-based facility shifted to today's workable hospital and community-based facility. I went from being extremely keen to have MS Neurologists on site in the community, to less so. I am now happy that the two are separate. It takes time for paradigm shifts to occur, and now I, too, am more patient. I would like to thank publicly, all the people involved in the above process for their efforts. Vancouver Island (approximately 700,000 people and 1,300 MS patients) has moved forward considerably in the last seven years. It is this Island's "struggle with change" that has moved me, a specialty physician, to write this book. My passion, providing health information to empower others with chronic illness, has improved my life, and I hope, the lives of others.

An MS Society should exist in your community; if not, look around and start one. Ideally try to start a group for those who have had MS long-term and also a group for the "newly diagnosed" and/or "newly accepting" of a diagnosis. "Newly accepting" includes those "out of the closet", which can be one to twenty-five years. We all benefit from the sharing of each other's experiences, contacts and networks. Many of us will not progress to walking assists or wheelchairs. Yet, the more we educate and understand each other, the more hope is truly possible. Certainly the bumps and knocks of our life experience are useful. Feelings of bitterness and hopelessness are temporary, so let's shorten them as quickly as we can.

Chapter 4

Income, Work or
Volunteer Activities

This topic will be very significant to many of us with MS. Job loss, job interruptions or reduced working hours can become a reality. The likelihood of recovery is reduced if we feel trapped by finances, bills and phone hassles with creditors. We know we have hit a wall when we are juggling bank overdrafts with credit card upper limits month after month. The buck inevitably and unhappily stops with us when we "rob Peter to pay Paul" once too often.

Financial issues were another major part of the illness crisis for Denise and I. We very nearly lost everything when my illness ended my anesthesiology practice, despite having a sizable income before diagnosis. After 30-90 days of no income, virtually all of us will hit a crisis. Our savings (RRSP's in Canada or RIA's in USA) went to paying acute debt (deferred taxes and emu farm expenses). Denise confessed that one of her greatest fears was, despite all our hard work and years of training, that we would be penniless and that she would be a poverty stricken widow. Loss of our primary relationship through death or divorce is all too common in MS or any major chronic illness.

Each of us must seek all the help we can in this tough, 1-2 year period when we progress from relapsing-remitting MS to secondary MS, or when we start with primary progressive MS. An MS expert at Scripps Clinic in San Diego, California diagnosed me with primary progressive MS. In reality, it matters little once you reach the progressive stage, whether it is primary or secondary MS. Treatments by traditional medicine are quite limited, and symptom management, or control, is the best they can do.

It is in this respect that we believe the individual or couple has to be especially proactive. We need to feel empowered, that we can control our own destiny. Without hope, deterioration can be rapid, severe and lead to depression, or institutionalization. In my experience, most people diagnosed with a significant degree of MS, will need to reduce their working hours or quit their job.

The road to financial stability in MS can be rocky and tortuous. Bureaucracy is tough to deal with when you are physically and mentally exhausted. The recurrent insurance forms still need to be carefully and meticulously done. Try to make it a game; if you take it too personally, the bureaucracy wins out. Most disability programs are full of detail and repetition which causes frustration. My advice is to get the very best advice you can. Often this means linking up with your local MS Society or Chapter. I had considerable problems with my application for disability. This was in spite of my time in family medicine practice and my having a conscientious and experienced Family Practitioner, Dr. Candace Cole. The bureaucracy pushed me to the limit, including nearly two years of waiting. In addition, I was finally advised that my case needed to be heard by a "tribunal" for a final decision. I searched for information and "team support". After four months, one week before the scheduled tribunal, they relented and agreed that I qualified for a disability pension. In retrospect, I wish I had looked for help sooner through our Vancouver Island MS Chapter, part of the MS Society of British Columbia, and part of MS Canada. You, too, will have a local, state or provincial, or national body near you. It is up to you to seek their help, online, in person or whichever way you can. This is one service at which they are good, because of their experience. You need their help So – ask for it!

The following includes a number of useful concepts anyone with MS should consider when applying for disability benefits.

Symptoms and disabilities are most accurately described as "those consistent with your worst days." Why? Because we have no control over what each day will bring!

Look for allies – those who have expertise in your community, one of the MS support groups or even the government. Your local MS society, especially a social worker, can point you in a good direction. My extremely supportive lawyer colleague wisely says, "Don't let those bastards grind you down, cause that's what they want to do!" In fact, bureaucrats are often rewarded for keeping or getting you off a disability payroll. Keep your long-term needs in mind and take it one step at a time.

Complete insurance or disability forms only when you are in your clearest thinking state. Denise and I have been supremely appreciative of the assistance of friends and their associates in this matter. If you quit on your valid disability application, then the bureaucrats win! The insurance companies would rather not pay out money. One to two years of economic hardship can turn into a decade, even a lifetime.

Positive work and income options are needed. If you are fortunate, you may be able to develop an ongoing, flexible relationship with your workplace. Beware of inner pride! Some of us with MS will not "take advantage", or "abuse" our disability. Please give your head a shake. Being diagnosed with MS is a life-altering experience. Acceptance of your diagnosis and taking control of your work, diet and exercise changes, and empowers you to make the best of your situation. Pride and the fear of "being treated with pity" are dangerous defence mechanisims. Take pride in what you can do, whether exercise, grooming or listening to a friend. Taking pride in your 'closet MS' secret, is dangerous, and can work to your long-term detriment. Denial of MS is no more useful than denial of a cancer diagnosis.

What options do we have regarding earning income? Usually we need to plug into a network of business associates or friends who still value our input. I was fortunate to eventually become the "world's expert" on emu oil. This gave me some self-esteem and made me feel needed once again. We need to find a niche for our passion or expertise. Think long and hard about this issue. Home-based businesses are more available today than ever before.

Today, Denise and I are passionate about educating and empowering people to eat right and be aware of the food supplements that are optimal for health. Fulfilling a niche as an educator is often possible. Distributing health or wealth information, tutoring and even direct sales are all niches for educators. The Internet is a new cornerstone for this option. The Internet, coupled with low telephone rates, increases our options of working solely from home, or at least part time, from home.

Please look at Denise's and my solution to find examples or choices for yourself. Consider your own knowledge and skills. We are now in the "information age". This creates a new business niche called "information entrepreneurs" or to use Robert Allen's term "infopreneur". This book is an example of our moving into this infopreneur stage. Our goal is to provide up-to-date health information for people with MS and other chronic illness. Chronic illness is increasing in many parts of the industrialized world. This self-published book is an important building block in our long-term financial security. Since I am unable to practice anesthesiology, I will take my "drug" expertise and apply it to food. Denise's dietetics training, her Masters in Nutrition, and her vast clinical experience, has helped me immensely.

My being diagnosed with MS has changed my perspective greatly. Flexibility and diversification are key. We have taken many personal development and training courses, primarily through a Canadian-based company, Peak Potentials (see Resources for internet links). Books, community resources, disability resource groups and even MS Chapters will enhance your awareness of options. Yes, you may be forced to create your own employment, so make it one you like!

If someone had told me I would be concerned about nutrition or personal training skills in my late 40's and 50's, I would have said, "Not bloody likely!" But, I would have been both wrong and shortsighted. I now believe Denise and I can help people more, with what we have learned together, than with my practicing medicine (Anesthesiology).

Certainly many of today's products are first available through direct sales, internet, mail order or networking companies. This makes sense, no matter whether it is a special food supplement, book, newsletter or health care product. This allows the client the option to "shop" or "sell" from home. These features dovetail well with many of us who are relatively "community" or "home" bound individuals. I believe this is particularly important for young, single parents, who are primarily women in their 20's, 30's and 40's, when MS peaks. So, please go to our website, not just to buy something, but also for ideas "outside the box", where you could work with us, for us or even emulate us. If the internet is not an option, send a letter or telephone us, using the contact information listed under Resources.

I firmly believe a home-based business can be a valuable option for many. What are some of the advantages of a home-based business? Firstly, many costs can be minimized. Secondly, some of your costs, such as office space, computers, utilities, telephone, internet, car and even clothing (especially dry cleaning) may be tax deductible, from earned or even other income. In Canada, for example, often six to eight thousand dollars per year may be reasonable to deduct from your "other" salary income, before paying your income tax. Denise and I first did this with our hobby farm project with emus. Denise was on salary, as a dietitian and so this helped reduce her tax bite because she had a home-based business. In fact, in Canada, you can barely afford not to have a home-based business, for this reason alone. The major requirement is that you must have reasonable expectation of profit within two years of start-up. I have watched vineyards and Christmas tree farms spin this out over seven or eight years.

Thirdly, start-up costs are usually reasonable. A package or business start-up kit is often available and can be acquired for less than a thousand dollars. Another business option is a franchise, or ready-to-go "cookie cutter" business. This, often, is considerably more expensive. Do your due diligence. Talk to friends or people you trust who can help you with this. Certainly our last three years of education, training and hands-on experience has allowed us considerable expertise in this area. Health information, and health products can be lucrative businesses as we baby boomers (born 1946 to 1966) age and move towards retirement. Most of us are seriously looking at staying healthy. Your venturing into this sphere can be as simple as joining Denise's team by purchasing a health product that you respect, or want to try. As with most things, you should first try a product. If it helps you, you are started toward success, as your personal story will mean a great deal to others. Personal care and beauty products have been successfully promoted in this manner when we consider such organizations as Avon or Mary Kay cosmetics.

Denise and I are most happy within health products. This encompasses our passions, our expertise, and now our successful personal story of recovery for each of us. We need new team players with us, in all regards. My experience with most people with MS is they have a zest for life and are great people to get things done. Movers and shakers, regardless of individual disability, are people we can work with. Your first step in due diligence might be as simple as listening to Denise and I speak, meeting us personally, or even via mail, telephone contact or email. Now is the perfect time for a home-based business to interact with others, even across long distances or globally.

Multiple sclerosis is a very common life challenge, which frequently occurs to men and women at the start or peak of their income generating ability. This certainly happened to me. However, Denise and I aim to turn this situation into a positive one.

Our wealth information training has taught us to work toward multiple streams of passive income. This could be as simple as a network marketing affiliation, owning a car wash or laundromat, or as complex as an ongoing newsletter and book on your expertise or passion. One example I recall hearing was of a man with twenty-years experience in selling and repairing kitchen fridges. He started an evening seminar on fridges to teach homeowners the nuances of what was available, and what might work best for them, their kitchen and their lifestyle. Subsequently, he became the number one fridge salesman and entrepreneur in that city or region. Another success story is a woman from Saskatchewan who solved a problem and then sold the solution. Her observation was that many newborn calves had their ears frozen during Canadian winters. Her "ear muffs for calves" became very popular among cattle ranchers and farmers alike!

Network marketing, especially with a unique or excellent product, has matured over the last three decades. In the 1960's, it meant buying and then selling a garage-full of soap. Then, in the 1970's and 1980's, it became a personal trust and relationship business for home and personal care products. By the 1990's and to date, this has matured further, with health and wellness products. The internet, inexpensive telephone and travel have permitted this burgeoning health and wellness industry to add unique products which require some education by experts. Both the envelope of whey protein isolate and the antioxidant scanner described in this book are two different companies that fit this health niche very well.

In today's world, network marketing, or direct sales, has many advantages. Besides low start-up costs, the people handling the sales (i.e. distributors) do not have to buy or carry an inventory of product. Instead, the distributor assists the customer in accessing product from the company, usually by use of a credit card. The product is then shipped directly to the customer's residence. The distributor is then responsible for follow-up with the customer. Income for the distributor is based on the volume of product purchased by customers. Income is also generated when the distributor recruits other people who become distributors. Communication today is fast and easy with the use of machines, cell phones, computers, conference calls, 3-way calls and couriers.

An important advantage of network marketing is the ability to generate more income than a regular job might provide. Hard work and building relationships can pay off in direct sales. Furthermore, network marketing allows for the leverage of time and the generation of a passive income. Passive income occurs as a result of training others to do the job (duplication). Passive income is income that is generated even when you do not actively work the business.

Another significant advantage of a credible, successful, well-established direct sales company is training. The men and women who work as independent distributors within these companies can train you. Corporate training is often available, as well. Denise and I still prefer the one-on-one or "kitchen meeting" training. This is people interaction at its best – problem solving, networking and emotional sharing of wisdom. Two of my best friends, Frank and Paul, are because of our involvement in a direct sales company. I mention this because men rarely develop close friends with other males. We need this, every bit as much as women.

Finally, in our era of big box stores providing many of our personal needs, there are still times we would like to speak or interact with a real person. If that direct sales or network marketing individual has developed trust in their relationships, and maintains that trust, it becomes a win-win situation. Furthermore, if one or more members of that individual's team has a high degree of credibility, this success or business opportunity is further enhanced. Denise and I believe women are best as network entrepreneurs. However, any of us can succeed if we develop trust and follow with our interpersonal skills rather than the "hard sell", often thought of, but now outdated.

If work in your regular area of employment is not possible because of MS, or if network marketing, infopreneurship, or other types of work are not options, then perhaps volunteering is. Many of us with MS volunteer our time, energy and wisdom to help others with MS or other life challenges. Scan your community for options to volunteer. There are many service clubs and non-profit organizations that are eager for help. Being a volunteer can be rewarding. Not only will you have the opportunity to discover new friends or develop new skills, but you will also benefit spiritually. Helping others is good for the soul.

In summary, there are a number of potential courses of action, despite a life altering illness. A time honoured quote would be, "When one door closes, often another one opens." Be creative, sincere and if need be, humble, to look for new solutions. Often volunteering in something you enjoy or believe in can be a great start. Similarly, if family or others offer to help, then create a way so that they can. This benefits both of you in the long term – health and/or financially. Learn all you can about your disability options, regarding pensions or tax deductions. Remember, knowledge is power. Finally, begin today, step-by-step, to create a new personal network. Any steps that you take will enhance your chances of recovery in mind, body and spirit.

Chapter 5

Caregivers At Home
And In The Community

Sometimes it is a matter of timing in a relationship with respect to who is the caregiver. However, with significant MS, the illness can dictate the need to receive and accept care. Denise and I have struggled with similar issues in our own relationship. My being a physician, or "caregiver" – especially in family practice, made this issue more clouded, not less.

My denial of my MS worked all right for a time. However, once the "wake-up call" became loud and clear, I had to "get it" and stop work. My stopping work greatly aggravated my self-worth. Over the years, as a male, I had defined my self-worth by helping those in my personal reach and practice of medicine. My self-esteem plummeted and finally said to Denise, "I am worth more dead than alive." Needless to say, this stymied Denise as to what to do or how to begin her role as caregiver to me, a person with MS.

Fear, and the uncertainty of what will happen in your life due to MS, are major complications. We are all a combination of personal circumstances and interactions. If you meet others with MS for the first time at a long-established support group, this can be a very negative and upsetting experience. Why? – Because we incorrectly assume that if most of these people are wheelchair bound, or are having trouble walking – then we will too! I still remember medical school when we were exposed to difficult genetic syndromes

39

for several hours a day, several days a week. What were my female classmates thinking who were pregnant at that time? "Will my baby be born with a birth defect?" It is very hard to keep our emotions and fears in a normal perspective, when personal experience strongly suggests otherwise. The ultimate fear of severe MS, how it will burden the family or others, greatly challenges the caregiver. This is why we wanted to include a chapter on this important issue.

Women are more often the caregivers, just as they are more often the ones raising children. However, 70% of those of us with MS are women. This, too, is a great challenge on a relationship when this "role reversal" becomes necessary. It also makes the sustaining or nurturing of the relationship with the caregiver, incredibly important.

Perhaps what I should be saying is that each caregiver and affected individual needs to take special steps to optimize or even survive his/her role. I believe, adapting to this physical and economic change is a key piece of the recovery and acceptance puzzle. In the following discussion we hope to outline some of the components that have helped us.

Firstly, when I was diagnosed, Denise's workplace had a modest but available Employee Assistance Program (EAP). This made several counseling sessions possible for us as a couple. Loss of job / health is one of life's greatest stresses and this counseling helped us verbalize and accept the change. I would suggest everyone seek out a similar option. As a self-employed physician, I did not have such an EAP option. If there is no EAP, look for other types of support – such as your local MS Society, family services or community groups such as a service club or church.

Secondly, we sought follow-up and received this from our Victoria-based MS Society, here in British Columbia, Canada. Our family met for 60-90 minutes with the Society's social worker to explore the impact my illness had on all five of us – Laura, Brian, Warren, Denise and me. I am usually pleasantly surprised when I see the depth of understanding that was possible with our three teenagers. Laura, our youngest, had to change schools because of our financial crisis. She did this willingly, without whining, complaining or fanfare. This was incredibly helpful to Denise and I. Our sons, Warren and Brian, were much more willing to help me once they understood that my irritability and short fuse was MS-based, and not just me, in the role of a father.

Thirdly, our local United Church minister followed our family closely with support in this time of crisis. I was listed weekly under "Prayers of Support" for more than a year. Now, I am more able to understand the significance of "universal consciousness" and support. It is an important part of the healing possible in the "mind, body and spirit" connection. Dr. Michael Greenwood discusses part of this in his book, "Paradox of Healing" which is listed in the back of this book, under resources. In addition, Larry Dossey, MD and Bernie Siegel, MD, in their books, go on to talk about the significance of prayer and caring.

Our ability to accept our own trials and forgive others, and ourselves is very important. Yes, I hung on to anger for many months, and still have some, eight years later. But, thankfully, I was able to let it go, for the most part. Some three years later, the person who was the source of my most painful personal interaction asked for my forgiveness before moving from our community. Denise and I attended the farewell for he and his wife. That particular occasion took considerable effort, but was a key part of acceptance and healing for both Denise and I.

Fourthly, there was family care giving challenges. My Mom and Dad already lived quite close by when I became ill. They were very active in giving their time, energy and even money when we were in sore need of all three. My parents' input, and a very supportive personal bank manager meant we did not lose our home and emu farm. Then my Dad was diagnosed with a lymphoma cancer six months after I was diagnosed with MS. This meant I needed to give back to him after six months of accepting support from him. It also eased tension between my Mom and Denise. Their efforts to help me sometimes collided, just as two strong wills on a similar mission, can do. Mom was now very committed to Dad's trials of radiation, chemotherapy and finally his slow, reasonably comfortable death at home.

In addition, this pulled my brothers and sisters back together in common support of my parents. This closeness had been very strained following my brother Stewart's death three years earlier. I believe we underestimate the power and significance of shared grief and circumstance. Births and weddings are ready markers for us, as are deaths and other crises such as moving, job loss, or health loss. Certainly life continues on around you despite your illness. I feel more in control of my own destiny now. It is wonderful to share this possibility with others, whether through this book or through health seminars.

Key issues for the caregiver are support and respite. Bonnie, the social worker of our Victoria-based MS-Canada Society, always includes one of her eight sessions with an emphasis on the caregiver. In this way, people in these sessions share their ideas, frustrations and even exchange emails or phone numbers. Hope for the future is very important for the caregiver as well. Whenever this is lost, it is a huge task to regain it. People can climb mountains, but rarely do if we tell them it can't be done.

Respite is an opportunity for a break away from "constant" caring. The more continuous (e.g. twenty-four hour) care is required, the more critical is the need for frequent breaks or respite for the caregiver. Often family or friends supply this. However, often this is impossible or not enough. Here, again, support from your MS Society individual can be very helpful in arranging this. The phrase, "All you have to do is ask." is not remembered often enough. It is our pride, the MS person's and/or the caregiver's that gets in the way.

I believe a humble sensitivity can help move mountains as it helps the human spirit immeasurably. If you like country music you may recall the line, "It's my belief, pride, is the chief cause of the decline of the number of husbands and wives". When one of a pair or family is stricken with chronic illness, this pride makes for a danger zone. Our ability to maintain close relationships, or reduce toxic ones, can have a profound influence on the health of both the client and caregiver. If the caregiver falters, or leaves, the client frequently needs institutional care. In multiple sclerosis, this very rarely permits the return of independent living.

Denise's Perspective:

The diagnosis of a chronic illness can put any person or family into a tailspin. Although I had worked in healthcare and had encountered many people facing a serious illness, I did not fully realize the ramifications. Personal experience is a great teacher. When Bill was diagnosed, it was almost a relief. He had been very short-tempered and on edge. Things just didn't seem right, but I chalked it up to a busy lifestyle. However, the level of stress had been gradually escalating in our family. It was good to be able to pin a cause to this stress, to help explain just what was going on.

Initially, I was too numb to deal with the diagnosis. I concentrated my efforts on just making it through each day. Bill spent a lot of his time sleeping, being totally exhausted and low energy. Farm chores and day-to-day family life consumed what energy I had. Some of my energy was also taken up by being a "peace keeper" or mediator when patience failed among family members. Bill's moods were volatile. I think that the emotional fallout of chronic illness is far more difficult to cope with than any physical changes that occur. Other caregivers dealing with family illness will no doubt identify with this.

In truth, I cannot recall many of the details of the first three years of Bill's illness. It was like I had plummeted down a black hole of despair. Bill was so sick and I felt there was not much I could do to make him better. I do know that I was angry and fearful, both destructive emotions. I was angry at an illness that took away Bill's ability to do work at which he was so very talented. I was angry at an illness that had come at a time in our lives that was happy and good. I could not understand the "why" behind the illness.

I was fearful of our now unknown future. As Bill's symptom worsened, I was fearful that he would lose his independence and become more disabled. Would I lose my husband, my soul mate? We were supposed to grow old together, enjoying our children as adults and grandchildren to come. It seemed like our social life had been reduced to people in wheelchairs, people who were becoming more and more disabled by this dreadful disease. I was fearful, as the bills accumulated, and no money came in, that we would lose our home. I was also worried about the impact on our three children. They had experienced Bill's mood swings and knew too well the tension in the household. There were times that I wanted to leave the chaos of our lives behind and escape to some deserted island.

I remember feeling very vulnerable at this time. Although I had worked hard in my profession, I had been assisting Bill with his bookkeeping, taking care of the family and the farm. I did not have a source of outside income. Fortunately, I was able to obtain work at the local hospital. This was important to me, because I knew that I could survive on my own, if that became necessary. It also really underscored the importance of maintaining professional ties and work affiliations.

I am glad that I persevered; I am glad that I weathered the storm. I am grateful that our children have also "hung in there". Gradually, as time passed, Bill seemed to get a bit better. The chaos settled down. The stress levels declined. It seemed like we were emerging from the long dark tunnel. We began to socialize more and didn't feel like we were in "survival mode" only. It became possible to envision a future.

What we experienced individually, and as a family, is no doubt similar to what many experience when a chronic or life-threatening illness strikes. Some of the things I found very helpful were the counseling sessions that Bill previously mentioned. These sessions gave me an opportunity to vent my anger and fears in a safe environment. I would encourage anyone struggling with illness and disability to seek help from a professional counselor. Church affiliation was extremely beneficial. The visits from people in our church and from our minister were very much appreciated, as were their prayers.

Support and assistance from friends was also appreciated. I am part of a women's group that meets to share stories and songs. I am grateful for the listening ears and compassionate support from this group.

I am also extremely grateful for the support provided by Bill's parents. The help they provided in so many ways, was invaluable. We feel blessed by the support and understanding of our three children. Without the love and support from these family members, and that of other family members, it would have been so much more difficult.

When reflecting back on the past few years, many thoughts come to mind. One is the importance of relationships, be they with family, with friends, or with the people we associate with in church, at the gym, in service clubs, or other types of groups. When the going gets tough, the support from these sources can make a difference.

Another realization is the importance of support groups like the MS Support Group that Bill has been involved in and the importance of umbrella organizations like the MS Society of BC and local chapters. So much good work is being done with fairly limited funds. Bill and I have supported these groups over the years since his diagnosis and we look forward to continued involvement. So, if a critical illness strikes your family, do seek out the local support groups. You will all benefit greatly.

Another reflection is the unpredictability of life and the ability to trust in a Higher Power. For a long time, I could not grasp why this was happening to us. I now believe that many things happen in life, which are not within our control, but are being orchestrated by a Higher Power. There are no coincidences in life. Bill's destiny was not to be an anesthetist; rather his medical training and skills have prepared him for the work he does now in educating others with chronic illness. He not only offers helpful advice, but he also provides people with hope for better health. Nor was my destiny to remain within traditional health care. I feel that my contribution now complements Bill's work and also benefits people in ways I could not have otherwise achieved. The world is full of endless opportunity—we look forward to the future with great optimism. We all need to trust that things will work out over time. Helen Keller's words seem especially appropriate "When a door of happiness closes, another opens; but often we look so long at the closed door that we do not see the one which has been opened for us."

Chapter 6

MS, Brain Fog, Depression, Cognition & Suicide Issues

The number one cause of death in people diagnosed with MS is suicide. Why is this so? We have already lost three very close friends with MS to this "loss of hope" endpoint. One friend was a successful professional, divorced twice since his MS diagnosis, who wanted out of life, before he got worse. He was pushing away his close relationships to distance himself from pity. As he moved toward despair, and lost hope of recovery, he sought death as his exit, while he was still physically capable. A second friend was a woman who had to leave work as MS had reduced her cognitive skills – gone was her ability to problem-solve. She was living evidence of how MS could severely limit the multi-tasking that modern life requires of us.

We now know the person most likely to commit suicide is the successful, determined individual. When they decide to take a course of action, they invariably, succeed.

The person afflicted with MS comes to personally understand the fragile ecosystem of the human brain. Fortunately, we have been able to learn some useful ideas and patterns that may help us regain and maintain hope.

Years of experience have shown that depression is more common with most any brain "injury" or illness. Other ones include not only stroke and brain trauma (i.e. head injury) but also degenerative diseases such as

ALS (Amyotrophic Lateral Sclerosis), Parkinson's and Alz-heimer's.

Fifty per cent of people diagnosed with MS will sustain a major depression sometime following diagnosis. Before the diagnosis, our risk is only 15%. Battles with depression can even appear prior to the diagnosis of MS. These episodes of depression can be treated with imipramine, our oldest (50-60 years) tricyclic antidepressant. Despite ongoing medication, I had one very bad time, 4-5 months after leaving work, when I got into a bottle of Scotch to "solve my troubles". Fortunately, son Brian put me to bed and removed the whiskey bottle. Depression and alcohol are a terrible mixture, as they can result in a downward spiral.

Excessive depression can lead to despair, and suicide can present itself as a solution. I have been very close to this state of despair. After more than a year of sliding downhill with my MS, the concept of suicide seemed a short cut. I am now incredibly grateful that Denise, Warren, Brian, Laura and my Mom, Alice, stuck with me. Once small steps of improvement occurred, the feeling of hope returned. This book is written to offer hope to people with MS or to those dealing with MS, or other chronic illnesses. It is our contention that once small steps of improvement can be made, the feeling of hope will return.

Some 65% of us with MS have the "invisible" but very real disability of cognitive difficulties. People with MS who experience cognitive trouble like to call this "brain fog". When I was further assessed at the Scripps Clinic in Southern California, I had to explain this more completely. To me, it is the relative inability to quickly solve a complex problem, or even prioritize well, a set of simultaneous problems. Once this MS neurologist had my cognitive skills evaluated, he realized this "brain fog" was one of my greatest challenges. Even now, three years later, I still have trouble remembering sequences, such as directions and have had to adapt around it. I have a great deal of empathy for others with cognitive troubles. Certainly, if depression is found on top of this, it seriously compounds the problem. The loss of concentration, associated with depression, can be minimized once the depression is treated. I work to optimize my day and minimize my stresses to reduce the risk of depression recurrence. Optimal MS recovery must include personal and peer support, in conjunction with Vitamin D, light therapy, psychotherapy and, when needed, antidepressant medication. The specter of suicide will always linger, so must be a consideration in times of high stress from any cause.

Research has shown "brain fog" tends to have no real or significant correlation to the physical disabilities of MS. (Cognitive troubles are an important component of my being unable to return to Anesthesiology.) Our woman friend, whom we lost to suicide, had a very responsible position and realized she could no longer cope with the demands of her job. Outwardly she seemed very determined to live her life to the fullest despite MS. However, we later learned from a mutual friend, that she and another MS sufferer had made a pact that if one of them lost their ability to control their mind's action, they would end their life while they still could. She hung herself at 49, in order to avoid her family seeing her in such a state. In the weeks before her death, she sought medical, psychological and psychiatric assistance. Tragically, she was turned down by the system in her city. Her story is another impetus for the writing of this book.

Solutions for depression increase as nutrition and health knowledge move forward. For example, reduced sunlight in fall, winter and early spring can lead to Seasonal Affective Disorder (S.A.D), a depressed mood. Light therapy can help S.A.D. The light used provides full spectrum illumination and is used 15-20 minutes daily. Light therapy can be a useful tool in beating back feelings of depression. A study done in Vancouver at the Women's Hospital revealed that this light therapy much reduced the incidence of post-partum depression. Other studies confirm the improvement in mood with light therapy. It is now understood that full spectrum light, bright enough, or long enough daily, raises melatonin production. Melatonin is the precursor, or building block, of serotonin and other neuro-transmitter substances in the brain.

A second, more recent discovery is that Vitamin D deficiency can aggravate depression. Recent data shows that reduced absorption occurs in some of us and we may need more vitamin D. Studies also show that many people in Canada have low blood levels of vitamin D as well as low intake of vitamin D containing foods. Further compounding the problem is the tendency for people to seek shade during the summer months, cover up exposed skin and apply sunscreens. Certainly, the RDIs of 400 IU for adults under age 70 and 600 IU for those over age 70, are not adequate (see Vitamin D chapter).

Counseling, grief work, and relationship enhancement can all help counter depression. First of all, we need to seek a higher power to forgive ourselves. Secondly, we have to learn to like ourselves for who we are, rather than rely on our work to define our self-worth. Often a full-steam-ahead, workaholic, Type-A person uses work done or achievements to maintain self-esteem. Again, this returns to the mind, body and spirit growth paradigm. Helpful books include those by Deepak Chopra, Michael Greenwood, Bernie Siegel and a host of others who all speak about this personal, yet very important personal journey. There is always life – but despair and depression can blind our hope.

We could all benefit from a recently published book "The Last Taboo – A Survival Guide to Mental Health Care in Canada", by Scott Simmie and Julia Nunes. The Canadian Mental Health Association of Canada describes it as "The best and most practical book ever written about mental illness and mental health in Canada". The association goes on to state, "The Last Taboo will do more than any previous publication to break down the fear and stigma surrounding people with psychiatric disabilities and encourage them and their families to take control of their lives." I believe a similar "control of their lives" is equally important for people with MS. Our depression and other mental neurological disabilities are often intertwined.

I like the book's candor, starting with the author's stories, progressing through the major frequency of mental disorder, its diagnosis and solutions – drugs and alternatives and suicide (the last taboo). I particularly appreciate their final chapter stressing the importance of "a home, a job and a friend". MS sufferers' needs are essentially identical. We humans are complex and spiritual beings and not, an island.

Simmie and Nunes point out "that recovery does not mean cure." "It is about living again, in a world beyond diagnosis. About regaining our rightful place in society." We suggest these powerful concepts are equally valid in a chronic illness, such as MS.

"Multiple Sclerosis, Diagnosis, Medical Management and Rehabilitation", edited by Jack S. Burk, MD and Kenneth P. Johnson, MD, contains a chapter on "Cognitive and Emotional Disorders", by Nicholas G. LaRocca, Ph.D. He writes of memory lapses, mood swings, grief and depression. Injury to the brain by MS leads to cognitive dysfunction. These can be further subdivided into such items as perseverance (refusal to give up; continued effort, especially under a handicap), deficits in executive functions such as planning, prioritizing and sequencing complex tasks, and reduced speed of information processing, reduced verbal fluency and spatial difficulties such as three dimensional or map reading tasks.

LaRocca continues to say that although severe clinical depression may be associated with mild cognitive impairment, there is little or no relationship between depression and cognitive deficits in folks with MS. Memory, both verbal and visual is the most common problem in MS. In addition, though short-term memory is usually spared, working memory, (i.e. the brief processing of information and temporary storage) is impaired. He states abstract reasoning and problem solving are also often impaired. Attention and concentration may be problematic especially if the topic is complex and sustained attention is needed. The above comments help describe our trouble with driving directions and problems following them.

In summary, LaRocca states MS may be thought of as undermining the overall organization of brain processes.

Some studies have found little or no relationship between cognitive deficits and physical neurological impairment or duration. "In contrast, many studies have found that patients with a progressive course are at greater risk for cognitive changes." Finally, cognitive changes may occur at any time during our MS and happen in both mildly and severely disabled individuals. In fact, persons with severe physical disability may be completely free of cognitive changes.

Chapter 7

Food Sensitivity and MS

In November 1997, I attended the MS Society of Canada's Conference in Vancouver for Complementary and Alternative choices for MS. This proved to be an important key to my modest recovery from MS. One of my sisters in Calgary had seen an ad or poster discussing the conference and alerted me. I had not heard anything about the conference despite living on Vancouver Island, only 2 hours from Vancouver. Of course, neither had I joined a local MS support group then. At this stage I believe I was using denial and withdrawing from others as a means of coping.

My family doctor, always very thorough and supportive, had probably told me about the local support group – but it went by me. In reality, most items went "by me", due to my loss of concentration and focus with MS. Approximately 60-70% of folks with MS have varying degrees of cognitive or "thinking" problems. At this time, I was not even reading the local newspaper, which announced the monthly MS support group meetings in my town. Actually, it was in registering for this Vancouver conference with MS Canada's, British Columbia provincial office, that the local MS Society contact was initiated.

I phoned the 1-800 number in Vancouver and explained I wanted to attend the MS conference. The woman in the office asked if I was a member of an MS Society or not. "No," I said, and asked what difference that would make. She explained it was $100 for physicians, but only $10 for members. Well, money was still very scarce at this time so I asked if I could join now and still qualify for the $10 conference fee. She agreed and wrote down my name, address and phone number so an employee of the MS Society of Vancouver Island could follow up on this. Indeed, it was meeting this Occupational Therapist for coffee 3-4 weeks later that started me on another key part of my journey.

I looked around the room at the Vancouver conference on the Saturday morning and was surprised at the room being nearly full with a wide spectrum of people. Many looked normal, while others looked challenged with a degree of disability. In reality, some of the "normal looking" had MS and others were family members or health care practitioners interested in MS (nurses, social workers, physiotherapists, occupational therapists, even an occasional MD).

The majority of attendees were young women, not surprising when 70% of people with MS are women and many of the interested health care practitioners are also women. Space and bathrooms were at a premium. About half of the folks in wheelchairs were men. By now I had learned that even though less men had MS, more of them are severely affected and often more rapidly progressive.

The presentations were varied, from medical descriptions of MS, to unique and particular therapies in smaller groups. Several people presented testimonials of their individual successes. I believe that these were especially useful to many of us with MS. Why? – because they were from the heart, and expressed "hope" to the audience: Maybe I can recover some as well!!

The symptom management sessions were helpful. One session presented healing and "retraining" or "recruiting" back-motor nerve pathways according to work by Meir Schneider. Another session and the most memorable for me, discussed the use of Chinese medicine, moxibustion, for pain and fatigue management.

However, the session that had the most impact on me long-term was related to the potential dietary triggers of multiple sclerosis and a discussion of the Stone Age or Paleolithic

Diet – the diet people had prior to 15,000 – 20,000 years ago. This was presented by Matt Embry, a young twenty-year-old man with multiple sclerosis from Calgary. I also met his parents who were with him. His mother had a degree in nursing and worked in public health. His father, Ashton Embry, who had a Ph.D. in geology and worked for the National Research Council, had done an exhaustive study of all the existing MS literature. His son had been diagnosed with severe MS at the age of 18.

From his family's research, Matt explained that diet was thought to play a key role in triggering and probably aggravating MS. He explained that grains and dairy products were often triggers of MS, through a process of "molecular mimicry". That is, a portion of the protein in the grain or dairy product was similar to that of the myelin surrounding the nerves. This protein portion escapes from the gastrointestinal tract and enters the blood stream. Because this protein is viewed by the body as being foreign, the body mounts a defense against the protein. Since the protein also looks like (mimics) the myelin protein, the body also attacks the myelin. Because of this error by the body, Matt explained that his family followed a reasonably restrictive diet with rice as the only grain, bananas, fish, white meat (chicken breast) and a few other foods. From information presented by Matt Embry, and from my discussion with his parents, I decided to look at the Stone Age or Paleolithic Diet.

Our current modern diet is a far cry from the Paleolithic Diet. At that time (prior to 10,000 years ago), humans ate 200 different "whole foods" per year. This included a very wide variety of fruits and vegetables, game meat and fish. Game meat and fish were sources of high quality protein and provided small amounts of saturated fat. It was extremely rare for people to have excess or even abundant fat, except for coastal fishing people. Grains were limited to small grass seeds, as this was prior to the Agriculture Revolution and grains had not yet become a large part of our diet.

Paleolithic people had a large intake of green vegetables and plants. This resulted in a large amount of omega-3 fatty acids being consumed. It is believed that we used to eat a much higher ration of omega-3 to omega-6 fats, 1:1 or 1:2. But today, as the dietary fat chapter outlines, many of us are 1:18 or 1:20 in our intake of omega-3s to omega-6s because of our high oil intake from corn, safflower, soybean oil and other oil crops.

Because omega-3 oils easily go rancid, they are not usually used in commercially produced foods. Consequently, omega-6 oils, which are hydrogenated or modified, are used in baked goods, most margarines and almost all fried foods. These modified oils have a longer shelf life and they do not taste rancid. However, they also contain harmful trans fats. We now know that trans fats are extremely harmful to our health and should be avoided!

Dr. Peter J. d'Adamo's book, "Eat Right for Your Blood Type" is a good start in understanding our need for dietary individualization. Certainly, determining blood type is one of the first steps when deciding upon organ transplants. A very good friend of mine who has 12 years of education in Food Science, is truly converted to the validity of food selection according to blood type. We should at least examine where we fit in. I am Blood Type A, which is suggested to be primarily vegetarian. Yet, I personally do better without wheat. That is a paradoxical statement for a Western Canadian prairie farm boy! Fortunately, Dr. d'Adamo's book provides sufficient detail for foods to be minimized in the diets of people such as myself with Type A Blood.

Other means to determine food sensitivities include VEGA testing and the ELISA blood test. In my first book I discussed the VEGA machine with modest enthusiasm. I now believe it is only a guide, and can lead to misinterpretation. Similarly, the ELISA blood test is not perfect either. This blood collection tests for antibodies to particular foods and in my discussions with many naturopaths, the testing labs are considerably hampered by available consistency of the base foods. In addition, occasional contaminants such as dust, herbicides and pesticides, or even peanuts, a common antigen, can skew the results incorrectly.

I admit I am weak with strict diets. I lasted only 5 weeks on the "Paleolithic Diet" outlined to me by the Calgary family. Next, my wife Denise and I set-up a progressive elimination diet for me at home. I carefully spent two weeks on it but learned nothing. I found this discouraging, as the "elimination diet" is considered the gold standard for "food sensitivity" by clinical and allergy research dietitians. In retrospect, I should have continued on the elimination diet for at least 4 more weeks.

Then, I got lucky, and discovered the primary trigger of my frequent migraines (80% of people with MS suffer from migraine headaches). By then, Warren, our eldest son, was attending university at the University of B.C. Like many college students, he had found the cheapest, acceptable beer with the highest percentage of alcohol of 7%, produced by a small brewery in Saskatoon. Needless to say, I was delighted when Warren brought some of this beer home one weekend. Finally, the shoe of who purchased the beer, was partly on the other foot!

However, much to my chagrin, whenever I drank one of the 7% beer, I would get a migraine headache. Ironically, I could drink two 5% beer, without a headache. Why the difference? Wheat was the answer. The extra sugars or carbohydrates in a beer made with wheat permit a higher alcohol content. Eureka! I gave up wheat thereafter. This included all modern wheat such as those in bread, buns, pasta, breakfast cereals and many processed foods. Denise taught me how to read food labels in order to eliminate wheat, wheat flour, wheat gluten, durum or even semolina from my diet. Wheat is by far the most common grain in Canada and the Northern USA. It is therefore an important component of many foods or snacks – including many chocolate bars!

I soon found if I cheated or made an error reading labels, I paid for it with a major migraine headache. This encouraged me to carefully select foods. As a bonus, I soon lost ten pounds (4.5 kgs) of weight! Many, many foods in North America contain some sort of wheat component.

I learned about spelt, an old wheat farmed until the late 1950's in Saskatchewan and now back in demand, especially in British Columbia. Kamut is also an old wheat (theoretically from King Tutankhamun's tomb of ancient Egypt, opened in the 1900's). Many of our friends on Canada's west coast, especially women, avoid wheat. They have found they feel better without wheat in their diet.

Similarly, when visiting health food stores in Kitchener, Waterloo (just northwest of Toronto), I learned more supportive data. The storeowner told me that many German and Austrian Europeans had immigrated to this region of Canada. However, most of them found they could not tolerate Canada's wheat bread or pasta. Consequently, there is a thriving spelt and kamut bakery and pasta niche in Kitchener-Waterloo. This trend towards the use of spelt flour is seen in other Canadian cities, including Vancouver, Victoria and Toronto.

The short story is, whichever grain is dominant in a society, a number of people will be "sensitized" to it. Hence the major grain sensitivity in Mexico is corn and in Asia, rice.

At the second British Columbia MS Society Complementary Medicine Conference in Vancouver in 2002, Denise and I learned more about why wheat and other foods were linked with MS. Our favourite speaker at that second conference was Dr. Lynn Toohey, of Colorado, USA. She has her PhD and has specialized in research of the Paleolithic diet. She explained about lectins, a small but important component that can trigger autoimmune diseases, particularly MS. Lectins are found in many foods including grains (i.e. wheat, barley), legumes (i.e. kidney beans, soybeans, peanuts), plants of the nightshade family (i.e. potatoes, tomatoes, peppers) and dairy. Lectins contain both protein and sugar. They are able to bind to the outside of a cell, including the lining of the gut, and cause biochemical changes in it. Thus, they can interfere with digestion and absorption in our gut. In the gut, they can damage the gut lining. Therefore, food proteins and lectins can then enter our bloodstream. These can then trigger autoimmune diseases.

In light of this, I then reduced my milk product intake, which seemed to further reduce my migraine headaches. I already knew I was lactose intolerant, so I had eliminated dairy products on an empty stomach unless I had lactase enzymes with me. I admit, I still cheat occasionally and eat ice cream and milk chocolate. I have never noted an issue with red kidney beans or soy products, but have minimized these, too. A further key point on diet that I have recently had confirmed, is the importance of digestive enzymes. Previously, I thought I only needed Lactaid with lactase, or Beano with some carbohydrate digestive enzymes. One or both of these would usually reduce my gastric hurry, diarrhea, abdominal cramps and excess rectal gas (flatus). I now know that a quality, general digestive enzyme containing amylase, protease, lipase and lactase is beneficial for me and many other people, especially as we age.

Denise had earlier taught me that fat is a common trigger of heartburn rather than extra stomach acidity. I agree, as a digestive enzyme before or with fatty foods protects me from heartburn. It is now accepted that acid reflux into the lower esophagus is usually due to a relative relaxation or opening of the lower esophagus sphincter (i.e. "valve"). Nearly all fat seems to loosen this physiologic valve with consequent heartburn. Hence, if the digestive enzyme lipase is used, heartburn is often avoided.

The further advantage of taking plant digestive enzymes with almost every meal is that there is a gradual reduction in acid secretion in the stomach, as we get older. The decrease in stomach acid begins at about 40 years of age and continues as we age. Taking digestive enzymes is very important to optimize our food digestion with enzymes secreted by the pancreas and gall bladder. Otherwise, we will not get the maximum benefit from our food and we might experience further unpleasant side effects. These include: diarrhea, rushing for a bowel movement, abdominal cramps and strong, often foul smelling gas per rectum (flatus).

A couple, originally from England, were delighted with this knowledge we shared with them. He had started to describe himself as the "Fart King of Vancouver Island". She had given up her favourite food, fish and chips, as she got either heartburn or abdominal pain whenever she ate them. Once they took two digestive enzymes prior to or with their meals, both troubles almost completely resolved. She can eat "fish and chips" as much as she wishes now!

I recently learned about another benefit of digestive enzymes when I was in southern Ontario. A friend had booked me for an appointment with a well trained and experienced live blood cell microscopist, whose background included over twenty years of clinical and research lab experience in a hospital. The day I visited this microscopist, my breakfast, two hours earlier, had been cheese/vegetable omlette and toast, with no enzymes. I was appalled at the incredible clumping (major and excess rouleaux formation) of my red blood cells. She then had me take 3 large capsules, removing the coating to speed the benefit, with 10 ounces of reverse osmosis water. She took another fresh sample of blood 25 minutes later. The microscope revealed an incredible improvement. I now had little or no clumping of my red blood cells! Recurrent clumping and reduced blood flow can definitely worsen your chances of a heart attack or stroke.

After this experience, I was deeply convinced about the benefits of digestive enzymes and will always add them to my regimen. If you are more than forty, or have MS, I would recommend a similar pattern. Europeans, especially Germans, have expounded on the value of these digestive enzymes. Wise use of such enzymes will likely pay for itself by further nutritive value absorbed from the food we eat. In addition, many unpleasant gut troubles may well be minimized, possibly even "leaky gut syndrome".

What is "Leaky Gut Syndrome" and why should we care? Leaky Gut Syndrome is thought to be due to local injury to the cells lining the small intestine. Keep in mind that our small bowel is 20-30 feet in length. This injury to the cells causes them to swell. Consequently, this reduces the "tight" contact between cells and allows undigested food particles to leak into the blood circulation.

Many things can cause local injury to the cells lining the small intestine. Major irritants are believed to be "food sensitive" or "allergic proteins" such as wheat or cow's milk proteins. Repeated insult from eating these proteins will worsen the gut "leakiness". Foods containing lectins can also damage the small intestine, leading to a leaky gut. Small pieces of proteins and lectins can now directly enter the bloodstream. The consequences of this ongoing, foreign protein "leak" through the gut lining and into the blood are several. Firstly, a set of white blood cells and their particular cell line is sensitized to the protein and increasingly expanded in numbers. Then, some secondary trigger, most likely viral, but possibly some other toxin (e.g. herbicide or pesticide), foreign protein, vaccination or something else of dietary origin causes a change in the white blood cells. Now this entire cell line of white blood cells is "permanently confused" and responds to a "similar looking" but ***different body protein***. If this protein is the lining of joints or synovium, we get rheumatoid arthritis. Similarly, if the protein looks like the protein lining of our myelin in our brain and spinal cord – we get multiple sclerosis. The term for some of our white cells attacking one of our tissues is molecular "mimicry".

One common group of drugs, the NSAID (non-steroidal anti-inflammatory drugs) such as ibuprofen, ASA, naproxen and diclofenac definitely can cause, or worsen, the "leaky gut syndrome". This is partly why they trigger gut bleeding in many of us. Local infections in the gut (bacteria from food poisoning or viral infections) can also cause a leaky gut.

Close cousins of the NSAID's are the COX-2 inhibitors, such as Vioxx and Celebrex. They, too, may have similar side effects. As a result, I avoid taking these medications and reach for acetaminophen (paracetomol in some countries), opiates (narcotics) or other painkillers. In addition, these same NSAIDs and COX-2 inhibitors are now considered responsible for slow healing in our bodies. Virtually all healing of skin, brain, joints and gut, have an inflammatory component to healing which is hindered and/or slowed down by this group of drugs. Sadly, repeated use of these drugs or the cortisone group, shorten our time before needing joint replacement or other surgical solutions, by reducing our body's ability to heal.

The other necessary component in multiple sclerosis is the "leaky blood brain barrier" associated with MS. Perhaps this foreign protein in the bloodstream reacts against these Blood Brain Barrier (BBB) cells similar to the gut lining. Now they have "holes" and it is through these that this sensitized white blood cell line passes to be able to attack the myelin lining the nerves in the brain and spinal cord. As alluded to earlier, wheat protein and milk protein are the two most likely triggers of MS that act in this fashion.

In reviewing the incidence of MS and geographical distribution, especially across the northern United States and Canada, questions come to mind. As one looks at the incidence of MS being greater in some areas, and not others, we need some additional reason to explain these differences other than just vitamin D and less sun exposure. I suggest that the high preponderance in the mid-West or prairies is the incredible intake of modern wheat and wheat pasta in this "bread basket" region. The second highest preponderance seems to occur in southern Ontario, Quebec, Niagara Peninsula or Wisconsin area. Perhaps this is related to the high milk and cheese production and consumption. As you reach the east coast, particularly Newfoundland, the incidence is somewhat less. Most people are of Celtic Irish heritage and from one of the genetic hotbeds of multiple sclerosis. Perhaps their reduced consumption of bread and dairy, relative to their prairie and Great Lakes counterparts, is partly protective for them. Similarly, their increased consumption of marine and fish oils may be further protective because of the increase of omega-3 fatty acids and Vitamin D in the diet.

In summary, food sensitivities and dietary components can trigger MS. Thus, current research supports eliminating wheat, cow's milk and lectins from the diet. I, too, recommend these dietary changes, but I do differ with respect to cow's milk. I believe dietary casein – the protein used in making cheese – should be eliminated. However, I also believe that a particular pharmaceutical or specialized whey protein isolate from cow's milk is beneficial. This particular whey protein isolate, which provides the body with bonded cysteine from undenatured whey protein, is discussed in further chapters on glutathione. In my review of data, my understanding is that a milk protein bound to milk fat (i.e. butyrophilin) may be a trigger of "molecular mimicry". The connection between butyrophilin and MS has been reported in the scientific literature. Because this specialized whey protein is fat-free, the risk of butyrophilin being present to trigger MS is remote. Furthermore, many people with MS have had considerable improvement in their symptoms from taking this specialized whey protein. This has also been noted by Dr. Toohey, a specialist in dietary triggers of today's autoimmune illnesses.

If you have MS or other chronic illness, I would encourage you to consider food sensitivities as being part of the problem. Try an elimination diet to determine which foods may be giving you problems. Eliminating certain foods from your diet can be challenging, but it just might help. Check with your Department of Health or medical center to find a qualified dietitian or nutritionist to help you with your elimination diet. You need to know which foods you can eat and which supplements to take so that your dietary intake is healthy and balanced in nutrients.

Chapter 8

Ongoing Total
Body Detoxification

Four questions that need to be asked are:

1. Do you believe our air quality is as good as it was 50 years ago?
2. Do you believe our water quality is as good as it was 50 years ago?
3. Do you believe our food quality is as good as it was 50 years ago?
4. Do you believe our environment quality is as good as it was 50 years ago?

Most of us would agree that none of these are as good as they were fifty years ago. On our journey to wellness, we should address this reality. In this chapter we will discuss the most natural, healthy and economic ways to do this. We will present alternatives to colon cleanses and intravenous chelation.

This chapter will again start at the cellular level, progress through tissues (i.e. lymph drainage) and then organs (i.e. liver, kidneys, lungs and skin) and finish with systems (i.e. digestive system and central nervous system, (CNS)). This permits us to do a comprehensive, step-by-step progressive, pleasant and affordable coverage of the subject.

To begin, we can be proactive toward what we breathe, drink and eat and the locations we choose to work and live in. Air quality is every bit as important as the others, and is one which we can neglect to our own peril. We now know that a child living on a busy street is more likely to develop leukemia than a child on a quiet street. The prime cause of the rise in leukemia is acute automobile, truck and bus exhaust. Residues from exhaust settle on sidewalks, roads and lawns. This is in turn deposited on floors, carpets and other surfaces that children play on. A youngster encounters this exhaust both from the air they breathe and through skin contact.

Skin absorption is an important issue with small children. This suggests the importance of minimizing children's contact with petrochemical products (not just gas or solvent), including petroleum jelly, (in U.K. white paraffin) and cortiscosteroid creams. Since we know that today's topical cortisones are stronger and that these steroids can have significant effects on bone growth plates, we should use instead, a topical, non-petrochemical product containing emu oil, shea butter or almond oil mixtures, whenever possible.

Other simple measures are the removal of shoes at the door and the change to indoor footwear. I believe the Japanese do this best. This measure alone greatly reduces our toxic load and protects a crawling toddler. In addition, we should favour hardwood, tile or linoleum and stay away from carpets, which have their own toxins.

Do you remember the "Mad Hatter" character in "Alice in Wonderland" by Lewis Carroll in 1865? The Mad Hatter was the partner of the March Hare at the Mad Tea Party. In "Alice in Wonderland", the terms, "mad as a hatter" and "mad as a March hare" were common and in use for thirty years already. Hatters (hat makers) really did go mad.

The most popular hat in the mid-1800s was beaver, but rabbit ones were cheaper. To toughen the rabbit fur fibers, a brush solution of mercurous nitrate was applied. Felt from the shaved fibers was immersed in a boiling acid solution to thicken and harden it. Unfortunately, the acid treatment decomposed the mercurous nitrate to elemental mercury which was breathed in and/or swallowed by the hatters. Recurrent exposure to the mercury (Hg) vapors caused mercury poisoning.

Victims developed severe and uncontrollable muscle tremors and twitching limbs, called "hatter's shakes". Other troubles secondary to Hg were distorted vision and confused speech. Severe cases developed hallucinations and even psychosis. Despite these serious side effects, the use of mercury in this way continued until 1941 in North America.

Does this story from history teach us anything? Yes, I believe it does. Removal of dental amalgams may be a useful piece of the "MS Recovery Puzzle". Similarly, if you are working in a dental practice on patients with mercury amalgams, and have MS, you should, perhaps, reconsider your pattern of practice. Newer options now exist. If your dental practitioner will not change, then you may need to change your dental practitioner. I appreciate both sides of this discussion exist, but you and I with MS have more reason for mercury anxiety than others – due to our neurologic illness. I debated whether I should have my mercury amalgams removed. When I met a bright, well-read, just retired dentist who had taught at three dental schools in Canada and the USA, I asked him. He answered that if he had MS, he would have his removed. This was good enough to have me proceed to do this. I believe it has helped – another puzzle piece.

The foregoing discussion may seem a bit overdone, but we now know more about exposure to toxins than we used to. It is sobering to think that today's teenagers, for the first time in recorded history, will not live as long as their parents. Each coming generation has more and more risk of autoimmune disease, obesity, diabetes mellitus (Types 1 & 2) and especially, cancer. As our water, air, diet and environment deteriorate, our illnesses increase. What we are exposed to and what we ingest have profound influences on our health, especially if they worsen oxidative stress. Most toxins do.

So, starting today, what can we do to reduce this ever-increasing toxic load? Dilution, dilution is the solution to pollution. For starters, we should increase our water intake, not pop, not juice, coffee, tea or alcohol, but water – aim for 8-12 glasses/day. Carry water with you (reverse osmosis is best to "clean it up") or buy bottled water from an ethically researched and documented company. Up to one-half of most bottled water is simply from the tap! Ozonated, spring water should contain no lead, mercury, herbicide, pesticide or petrochemical contamination. Dechlorinate your water at the tap with reverse osmosis, a carbon filter or at least a filtering pitcher, or leave water standing overnight before drinking to allow the chlorine to evaporate out (if it works for exotic fish it may help you, too!). It has been reported that over 60,000 chemicals have been found in our water supply. Over the course of a lifetime, we will ingest about 450 pounds of sediment and metals from our drinking water. Hopefully these statistics will encourage you to seek out purified drinking water.

Secondly if you need coffee or tea to survive, go organic, and prepare them with purified water. Why? – because more weed and insect sprays are used on growing coffee and tea plants than any other agricultural product. Sure, you can bend any of these suggestions if you wish – it is your journey. If you are uncertain and need reinforcement about the fact that "we are what we eat", watch the documentary film "Super Size Me." This movie has had more impact on the fast food industry than anything else to date. One major hamburger firm is already discontinuing the "super size" policy completely.

Thirdly, pay attention to and minimize your "empty", quick sugar calories. Reduce all pop and all juice cocktails, beverages and punches – these are primarily fructose, sucrose and water. Look for juices that are made from 100% fruit juice. Artificial sweeteners are not recommended. If you have a major sweet tooth, learn about stevia, a natural sweetener. Marketing companies have become very skillful in their approach to advertising and can seduce you into purchasing food products that not only have little nutritive value, but that can actually be detrimental to your health. Cigarette and alcohol companies have long understood these marketing principles.

You will soon discover that part of cleaning up our bodies is easily done by changing what we put into it. Refusing mercury amalgam dental fillings, or having old amalgam removed, will gradually decrease your toxic input. Similarly, by moving to an area with pristine air, clean water and good soil, great benefits can be realized immediately. Not all these choices are necessarily affordable, of course, but do what you can; it will not only gradually make a difference, but it will also strengthen your sense of being in control.

Denise has found in her work with clients of all ages that our parents' generation was the one which ate the best, with fresh, prepared whole foods. This is not because they had more income, but because they had better eating habits and many had retained the practice of having a vegetable garden. Today, many of us can improve our own habits with the help of community kitchens, food co-ops and private gardens. Alternatively, develop a relationship with a farmer/farmers you trust and respect. "Closer to home" - eating means more variety (seasonal), fresher produce and more control of how your food is grown.

What would be another method of cleaning up our bodies? The answer is more fiber. Soluble and non-soluble (ground flax contains both) will "scrub" your intestines, and help eliminate toxic wastes excreted by the liver into the bile, including the "bad cholesterol", LDL. Cooked legumes and whole grains are other excellent sources of fiber – but not wheat, barley or rye if you are gluten sensitive (celiac disease). Fresh fruits and vegetables are very good. Consuming wholesome food is, by far, preferable to cleansing regimes which bubble air, ozone, coffee, water, saline or x-ray dye up our butts, but this is, of course, a personal decision.

Should juice or water fasts be considered? If you want to go this cleansing route, take some time off for yourself. We have a physician cousin who died of a heart attack while working hard breaking-in horses and at the same time being on a 3-day fast. Doing "one thing at a time" will be difficult for those Type A workaholic types – some of whom have MS.

What supplements can assist this detox and body cleansing approach? Fresh water, fruit and/or vegetable shakes or smoothies and foods containing plenty of fiber should be among your first choices. "Fiber cookies" are one easy option. The multivitamin, multimineral, combined with Vitamin D, calcium and magnesium will also contribute to the cleansing process. Boosting our endogenous antioxidant, glutathione, inside the cell with a very good whey protein isolate, high in bioactive cysteine, will have a profoundly beneficial effect.

Glutathione is the number one molecule for detoxing or removing almost all drugs, heavy metals (Hg, Pb, Cd – Mercury, Lead and Cadmium), petrochemical residuals, tobacco-triggered free radicals, tar, and most herbicides and pesticides. Glutathione (glue-the-tie-on) is, without question, our optimal and cheapest detoxification ally. Water would be the only exception to this.

Dr. Gustav Bounous, Dr. Patricia Kongshavn and Dr. Wolf Dröge have all documented the health benefits of taking whey protein isolate (bioactive cysteine), an essential building block of our body cells. Look for these envelope pouches of fine white powder (see **www.emu.ca** for resources) made from cow's milk. In reality, any mammalian milk will have the same effect, and the very best of these, of course, is fresh human breast milk. However, as adults we do not have access to this option!

Those of you who are great fans of the Paleolithic or Stone Age diet, will no doubt feel this is blasphemy for someone with MS. All mammalian milk contains butyrophilin, and butyrophilin is a probable trigger for molecular mimicry, causing our own white blood cells (immune response) to pick on the myelin sheath around our nerves in our brain and spinal cord. However, this particular whey protein isolate, providing bioactive cysteine, is completely defatted and all the casein protein is removed as well. In most, but not all cases of milk sensitivity (allergy), the casein (cheese) component is the cause thereof. Only one in 100,000 will be allergic to this very clean, whey protein isolate. In addition, 99% of the lactose, the sugar in the milk, is removed. This means most people should have no problem, except for those who are extremely lactose sensitive. If you are lactose intolerant, take a supplement with the whey or a quality plant digestive enzyme, which will include lactase.

Further light on the milk sensitivity issue is found in a research paper by Drs. Toohey, Smith and Hickey published in April 2000 in the British Journal of Nutrition. We had the good fortune of hearing Dr. Lynn Toohey speak on this issue in Vancouver in 2002. She outlined the three most common triggers of food sensitivity and potential causes of auto–immune diseases such as MS or rheumatoid arthritis. The three common triggers were lectins from wheat, red kidney beans and casein. In personal discussion with Dr. Toohey later, she indicated that the primary problem was from the casein in cow's milk, not the whey.

Let us turn now to the subject of detoxification. Heavy metal poisoning is generally treated by administering chelation, intravenously or orally. One excellent example of oral chelation is the use of the whey protein isolate which provides building blocks for glutathione. This is explained more fully in Chapter 11 on glutathione.

However, there is an alternative method of detoxification that can be used: the infrared sauna. These small (2-4 people) sauna units, for home or shared use, emit radiant heat in the form of infrared energy. This means that radiant heat travels from the source to your body without having to heat the air in-between. Our sun produces most of its energy in the infrared segment of the light spectrum in the 7-14 micron range (a micron is 1/100,000 of a meter).

Our own body tissues produce infrared energy to keep us warm and to repair tissue. Our bodies radiate infrared energy through the skin at 3-50 microns, with the greatest output being 9.4 microns. For example, the palms of our hands emit infrared energy between 8-14 microns. Palm healing, an ancient tradition in China for 3,000 years, is also employed by yogis in India.

Dr. Tadashi Ishikawa, of Fuji Medical Research and Development, received a patent for a zirconia ceramic infrared heater. Only medical practitioners in Japan were able to use these infrared thermal systems, for the next fourteen years prior to 1979. They were then released for public use and have been sold in North America since 1981. Infrared heat has been used for many years to warm newborns and post-operative patients. Our own personal infrared sauna is made of red cedar from Canada's west coast and the Japanese technology mentioned above (see Resources at the back of this book or go to www.emu.ca).

A conventional sauna relies on an indirect means of heat (convection and conduction). Traditional saunas operate at 180-235 degrees Fahrenheit, whereas infrared saunas operate between 50 and 125 degrees Fahrenheit, which is 10-60 degrees Celsius. Hence, in an infrared sauna, you are able to breathe cooler air while at the same time feeling warmth. This is welcomed relief for the "cold, cold hands and feet" symptom of people who have MS.

Over the last 25 years, primarily Japanese and Chinese researchers have completed extensive research on infrared heat treatment. Their findings support the health benefits of infrared therapy as a method of healing. Over 700,000 infrared thermal systems have been sold in the Orient alone, and some thirty million people have received localized infrared treatment worldwide. In Germany, physicians have used whole-body infrared therapy for over 80 years. The wide-spread use of infrared heat and its consequent acceptance by Health Canada and the FDA in the United States, strongly suggests that its use is safe.

Now that we have established safety, what might infrared sauna therapy do for those of us who have chronic illnesses, especially MS? One benefit for MS folks is the use of infrared heat to produce cardiovascular conditioning. "Regular use of a sauna may impart a similar stress on the cardiovascular system as running or jogging, and its regular use may be as effective a means of cardiovascular conditioning and burning of calories, as regular exercise." This quote is from 7 August 1981, issue of the Journal of the American Medical Association.

No doubt some of you are wondering, "What if my MS and I cannot tolerate heat?" These individuals should move forward slowly and gradually with time and patience. An infrared sauna makes it possible for people in wheelchairs and those who cannot follow an exercise/conditioning program, to achieve a cardiovascular training effect. Initially, you can leave the sauna door open. This minimizes the ambient heat, while the infrared still penetrates to do most of its good. We now know that heat worsens symptoms of most CNS illnesses, including stroke and MS. However, most symptoms subside once cooling to normal temperature occurs.

In addition, nerves that have lost their myelin are particularly sensitive to heat – that would include MS! This may explain why some 70% of MS patients are very heat sensitive. I was, but am happily less so now.

Why would we consider infrared therapy? It ties in, in three ways. Firstly, the improved blood flow stimulates healing in all parts of the body. This includes our skin, brain and spinal cord. Secondly, the caloric consumption controls weight gain. Guyton's Text of Medical Physiology states that one gram of sweat uses up 0.586 calories. The Journal of the American Medical Association citation (7 August 1981) goes on to state, "A moderately conditioned person can easily sweat off 500 grams in a sauna, consuming nearly 300 calories —- the equivalent of running 2-3 miles. A heat-conditioned person can easily sweat off 600 to 800 calories with no adverse effects. While the weight of water loss can be regained by rehydration, the calories consumed will not be". Hence, the infrared sauna can help us with both weight control and cardiovascular conditioning.

Thirdly, detoxification is accomplished through sweating (perspiration). The infrared heat penetrates three to four centimeters (1.5-2 inches) beneath our skin. Our fat layer is usually here and so the increased circulation caused by the infrared will help the whole body to detoxify. Remember to replace your minerals too, especially sodium and potassium. Drink lots of water!

In summary, detoxification is achieved in many different ways. It is up to each of us to work out the best and most affordable option. Some of us do not handle heat well, so these folks must start slowly and carefully and should not think about making a sauna purchase before being totally comfortable with it. Exercise, discussed in another chapter on movement, is also a superb way to detoxify through sweat produced. Do exercise, but begin slowly, until you have built up tolerance. Careful detoxification with the whey protein isolate is an option for almost all of us. Ample water intake should be emphasized. Remember, "dilution, dilution is the secret to pollution!"

Chapter 9

Vitamins & Minerals – Supplementation for Optimal Health

Nutrition supplementation has become a burgeoning industry. Why has this occurred? We believe it is a shift in people's mindsets. Many of us, especially the well-informed, are now aiming for wellness and optimal health. It is now felt that 75 or 80% of our chronic health problems are nutrition based. In this chapter we outline three food pyramids to permit readers to see how we should be changing the emphasis from disease to wellness. The RDA (Recommended Dietary Allowance) background is next. Following this is a summary of the vitamins and minerals and other supplements our bodies can benefit from.

First, the three different food pyramids (See Figure 1-1). The "Official" USDA (United States Department of Agriculture) Food Pyramid, revised in 1996, outlines what to eat from each food group to be healthy and reduce risk of disease. Because of a concern that high fat diets cause cancer, heart disease, obesity and other diseases, the pyramid focuses on reducing dietary fat. It then encourages people to eat more carbohydrates from the breads, cereals, rice and pasta. However, in consuming a low fat, high carbohydrate diet, North Americans have continued to gain weight and develop more chronic illnesses than ever before.

In January 2005, new dietary guidelines for Americans were released. The new guidelines place a greater emphasis on reducing caloric intake for weight control and increasing physical activity (60-90 minutes daily). People are encouraged to get all of their nutrients from food. The dietary guidelines also identified that certain population groups should have a vitamin supplement. These include people over 50 needing vitamin B-12, either from fortified foods or a supplement and elderly people or dark-skinned people needing supplemental vitamin D. At the time of the writing of this book, a revised food pyramid had not yet been released to reflect the new dietary guidelines.

The "Mediterranean" Food Pyramid is from a cultural group that has less heart disease than we have in North America. The greatest change here is the emphasis on olive oil, a monounsaturated fatty acid.

The third and perhaps ultimate is the "Optimal Nutrition" Food Pyramid. It is designed by Roy Walford in his book *Beyond the 120 Year Diet.* All three pyramids are shown on the page opposite.

Walford has shifted fruits, vegetables, beans, and nuts to the anchor or dominant position. The diet should emphasize these foods. Carbohydrates are assigned a position on a glycemic index (or GI). The Glycemic Index is the ranking of different dietary carbohydrates on their ability to raise blood sugar levels. For example, boiled potato has a glycemic index of 88. This means that it is easy for the body to digest the potato and convert it into blood sugar. Chickpeas have a glycemic index of 28. Because of the fiber and other nutrients in the chickpeas, it takes longer for the carbohydrate to be released as glucose or blood sugar. Foods that are low in *complex* carbohydrates and high in *simple* carbohydrates, like cornflakes and sweet donuts, would be assigned a high GI. Foods like broccoli, apples, "grainy" whole wheat bread, and brown rice would be assigned a low GI.

One concern with high glycemic foods is their ability to cause a rapid and high increase in insulin in the blood. This is the body's way to lower blood sugar. However, blood

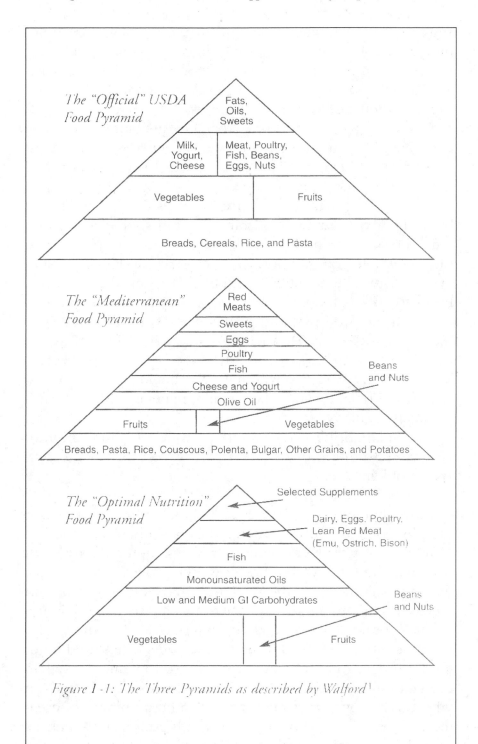

Figure 1-1: The Three Pyramids as described by Walford[1]

sugar levels may come crashing down, triggering a feeling of hunger and leading to overeating. In some people, especially when weight is a problem, the body develops insulin resistance and blood sugar and insulin levels remain high. The blood sugar is then directed into fat stores. You should eat foods with a low Glycemic Index so that 1) your blood glucose is controlled, 2) your cholesterol level is controlled and 3) your appetite is controlled. This in turn will lower your risk of heart disease and type 2 diabetes.

The vast majority of carbohydrates consumed should be in the low to medium GI range. Avoid simple sugars and refined foods. Reach for vegetables and fruits with your meals. Choose whole grains, whole grain products and lentils whenever you can. Remember, though, that using the Glycemic Index to choose foods is only one strategy for healthy eating.

In the food pyramid, Walford also puts selected supplements at the top. He recognizes many or most of us are unable to obtain all of our body's needs from food readily available to us. We agree with him. We should all eat according to his food pyramid and take vitamin, mineral, and other supplements regularly.

Finally, it takes five to six times as much nutrition to *reverse* a condition that's already in place as it does to *prevent* problems.

Genetically, humans are "old" beings; we probably haven't changed for hundreds of thousands of years. Our diet, by comparison, has changed drastically in just the last 10,000 years with the agricultural revolution, the discovery of fire, and the fact that we are now living on the majority of the earth's surface. All these changes have an impact on our dietary requirements and on what our dietary intakes should be. It is thought that 10,000 years ago, over the course of a year, we ate some 200 different seeds, nuts, fruits, and other foods. Today, we would be hard pressed to name more than 20 major foods in our diets. Most of these are based on wheat, rice, soy, corn, milk products, and a number of common vegetables— especially in North American—such as peas, beans, carrots, and corn. Further limiting variety is the fact that we can get most foods all year long by importing them from elsewhere. This often results in our eating a single variety of fruit or vegetable (for instance, only iceberg lettuce or Granny Smith apples).

All of these factors have made a difference. One of the other features of our modern life is that we have moved to more temperate climates, that is, further away from the equator. This has impacted on us as well, because most of us now live in areas where we can't make much vitamin D from the sun.

Dietary Reference Intakes
(Formerly "Recommended Daily Allowances")

Both Health Canada and the Food and Nutrition Board of the Institute of Medicine have led the development of nutrient recommendations in North America. Over time, these have become almost sacrosanct. The knowledge base for these nutritional estimates was based on six criteria:

1. The amount of the particular nutrient that healthy people consume.
2. The amount needed to avoid a particular disease (e.g., scurvy was very common and the recommended daily allowance of vitamin C is enough to prevent scurvy).
3. The degree of tissue saturation or the adequacy of body function in relation to that nutrient intake.
4. Nutrient balance studies that measure nutritional status in relation to intake.
5. Studies of volunteers experimentally maintained on diets deficient in a nutrient, followed by their improvement, or signs of deficiency going away, when a certain amount of the nutrient is re-supplied.
6. Extrapolation from animal experiments in which deficiencies have been produced by exclusion of a single nutrient from the diet.

From 1997 to 2002, a joint committee of experts from Canada and the United States collaborated to produce the

Dietary Reference Intakes (DRIs). The DRIs consist of 4 types of nutrient recommendations for healthy individuals: adequate intake (AI), estimated average intake (EAR), recommended dietary allowance (RDA) and tolerable upper intake level (UL).

When insufficient scientific information is available for a particular vitamin or mineral, adequate intake (AI) is determined. The AI is based on the approximate intake of a nutrient by a group, or groups, of healthy people. For example, the AI for adult men for manganese is 2.3 mg per day. For adult women, the AI is 2 mg per day.

The estimated average requirement (EAR), is the average requirement of a nutrient for healthy individuals. The EAR is the amount of a nutrient which would meet the needs of 1/2 of a given healthy population. Thus, EAR should only be used when assessing the nutrient adequacy of populations, not individuals.

The new RDA is the amount of a nutrient that would meet the requirements of 97-98% of healthy individuals. The RDA then becomes the goal for intake for individuals. It is important to remember that nutrient needs change throughout our lifetimes. What is needed for a child might be very different than that needed for an adult over 70. For example the RDA for folate is 150 ug/day for children ages 1-3, while the RDA for individuals aged 14 years and older is 400 ug/day.

Tolerable upper intake levels (ULs) have been established to reduce the risk of toxic effects from over-consumption of nutrients. The UL is believed to be the highest level of a nutrient intake that is safe for the specified group. It is felt by some that the range between the RDA and the UL may represent nutrient intakes that may promote health or prevent disease. Some scientists, health practitioners and nutrition experts disagree with the RDAs and ULs, and recommend even higher levels of nutrients for disease prevention and treatment of diseases. These higher levels would be considered a "therapeutic" level and would require ongoing supervision and counsel by the practitioner.

Since 2000, two very amazing developments have

occurred with respect to nutrition recommendations. Firstly, more traditional organizations began to recommend vitamin/ mineral supplementation. In 2000 and again in 2005, the United States Department of Agriculture (USDA) Dietary Guidelines for Americans recognized that some people need a vitamin/mineral supplement to meet specific nutrient needs. The American Dietetic Association has also adopted a policy statement addressing the use of nutritional supplements for some individuals. We applaud the AMA (American Medical Association) publishing in their Journal in 2002, that most Americans would benefit with a daily multi-vitamin/multi-mineral supplement. Many nutrition researchers, scientists and health professionals have been advocating vitamin/mineral supplements and other dietary supplements for quite some time. As science continues to shed light on the roles of nutrients and the optimum amounts and combinations for health and disease prevention, recommendations for dietary supplementation will continue to evolve.

The second development was the July 2002 Scientific American article by Walter C. Willett and Meir J. Stampfer, professors of epidemiology and nutrition at the Harvard School of Public Health and professors of medicine at Harvard Medical School. They set out to improve upon the United States Department of Agriculture Food Pyramid. Their New Food Pyramid is even more forward thinking than Walford's. In their "New Food Pyramid", Willett and Stampfer distinguish between healthy and unhealthy fats and carbohydrates. Healthy fats include liquid vegetable oils such as olive, canola, soy, corn, sunflower and peanut. Trans fat does not appear in the Pyramid. Healthy carbohydrates include whole grain foods such as oatmeal and brown rice. Willett and Stampfer recommend avoiding refined carbohydrates, butter and red meat. The New Food Pyramid features multivitamins for most, and alcohol in moderation. In addition, they included *daily* exercise (walking or running) on the base of the pyramid. The New Food Pyramid represents advanced thinking. Unfortunately, not all of us, including health care professionals, have accepted these wise changes – in our opinion.

We certainly advocate a healthy diet, based on whole foods, fresh foods and natural foods, preferably organic. We advise that people reduce their consumption of processed, packaged and commercial foods. This will help them avoid excess salt, sugar, fat and trans fat, all known to impact negatively on health. In addition, these foods usually have higher levels of preservatives and additives. They often provide fewer nutrients and more calories. However, as previously mentioned, it is increasingly difficult to get all of the nutrition we need from food alone. The following are reasons for supplementing with vitamins, minerals and other dietary supplements:

1. Crop nutrient losses: Our soils are becoming depleted of minerals, leading to a reduced mineral content in many crops. According to one study, 6 minerals are reduced by as much as 76% in the last 50 years. Another study by the University of Texas in 2004 reported a 38% decline in riboflavin (B vitamin) and a 20% decline in vitamin C as well as decreases in protein, calcium and phosphorus in 43 common garden crops.

2. Poor digestion is common among the elderly. Reduced gastric juices, lack of friendly gut bacteria, and stress can all impair digestion.

3. Microwave cooking causes changes in the food and alters the nutrition provided by the food.

4. Food storage can reduce the nutritional value of our food, especially fruits and vegetables. The average distance food travels from field to table can be as much as 1000 miles.

5. Food restriction because of weight loss diets, food allergies or food avoidance can result in poor nutritional intakes.

6. Poor lifestyle habits such as smoking, alcohol and caffeine can replace important foods, interfere with the absorption of nutrients or lead to nutrient loss from the body.

7. Stress, either physical or emotional, increases the body's need for vitamins, minerals and other nutrients.
8. Nutrient imbalances can impair how the body uses nutrients. No one nutrient can do the job alone. The body relies on a network of nutrients to keep healthy. Therefore a balance of nutrients is needed.
9. Variances in the nutrient content of foods.
10. Food selection can impact the nutritional value of a person's diet. If only a few different foods are regularly eaten, then the types and amounts of vitamins, minerals and other valuable nutrients will be low.

Listed in this chapter are the "official" RDA or DRI (daily recommended intake) levels of several important vitamins, minerals and other nutritional supplements. Listed below the RDA/DRI is the supplementation level we suggest. These amounts are *total* daily amounts. In many cases we also list a "treatment" level, which will apply to some individuals.

National surveys indicate that about half the population uses dietary supplements. Those that use supplements tend to be healthy people with positive attitudes about their diets and their health. Surveys have shown that the use of supplements by health professionals (including physicians, dietitians and pharmacists) is high. People who use supplements often have healthy diets and have healthy lifestyle habits, such as exercising and not smoking. Supplements **should not** be an excuse to eat poorly, skip exercise and neglect other healthy habits. Rather, supplements can be a form of "health insurance" toward good health. A healthy diet supplies thousands of other vital components needed for health, such as fiber, essential fats, minerals, antioxidants and phytonutrients.

Choosing a supplement can be difficult. The supplement market is a billion dollar industry with hundreds of companies producing a confusing array of bottles and potions. How to choose? The Council for Responsible Nutrition, which represents leaders in the supplement industry, proposes a "Dietary Supplement Pyramid". This gives advice on which vitamins or minerals are important to supplement. At the bottom of the pyramid is a multivitamin/mineral with 400 mcg folic acid. There seems to be a greater likelihood of benefit and no harm from a daily multivitamin/mineral for adults that meets the RDA.

Thus, a multivitamin with minerals should provide 100% of the Daily Value for all or most vitamins and a number of minerals. Most vitamin/mineral supplements will not be able to provide the full RDA amount of calcium. This is because calcium is needed in a large amount and is a bulky nutrient. Some calcium may need to be taken separately. A multivitamin with minerals can fill nutrient gaps, protect health and reduce the risk of disease. The bottom of the Supplement Pyramid should also include a source of omega-3 fat. Chapter 14 outlines the importance of the omega-3 fats.

The next level of a Dietary Supplement Pyramid would include extra calcium (1000-1500 mg for bone health) and vitamin D (1000-4000 IU) for bone health and prevention of autoimmune diseases and many cancers). The third level would include antioxidants (vitamin E 400 IU, vitamin C 100 mg, lutein, beta-carotene, and selenium) for cell protection and repair. At the top of the pyramid are supplements for special needs such as vision, healthy heart, joints, menopause and sports. The flag at the top reminds us that herbal supplements, which have a long history of use, can be used for many purposes.

Now that you have an overview of supplements, what are the criteria for judging among the several hundred thousand brands of vitamin/mineral supplements? One option you have as a consumer is to call the company directly. Some of the questions you can ask are:

1. does the company have its own research scientists?
2. does the company own farms that grow plants?
3. does the company do its own testing for quality, strength and purity?

4. does the company do clinical trials on their products?

A "yes" answer to these questions indicates a good nutrition company. Another option you have is to consult nutrition experts who have had experience with a variety of products. They will know which ones have a proven track record and which ones are perhaps not so good. Also, try to determine that the supplement:

- uses exclusively natural vitamin E containing a mixture of tocopherols
- uses optimum amounts of antioxidants: 100-400 IU vitamin E, 200-500 mg vitamin C, 5000-15000 IU beta-carotene, and 70-200 mcg selenium
- uses optimum amounts of bone nutrients: 500-1500 mg calcium, 210-700 mg magnesium, 200-800 IU vitamin D and at least 1 mg boron (40 mcg vitamin K allowed in the US, but not in Canada)
- uses optimum amount of B vitamins involved to lower homocysteine levels and reduce heart disease: at least 200 mcg folic acid, 1.5 mg vitamin B-6 and 2.4 mcg vitamin B-12
- provides significant amounts of carotenoids such as lutein and lycopene.
- Provides significant amounts of flavenoids from many sources i.e. quercetin, isoflavones, grape seed extract.
- Uses well-absorbed, bioavailable sources of trace minerals (chromium, copper, manganese, iron, zinc, etc). Check to see if the minerals are chelated. (chelated minerals are bound to protein and are easier for the body to absorb.) To check for chelation, look for the following words on the label: zinc as zinc chelate; magnesium as magnesium chelate, etc.
- Capsules should dissolve within 30 minutes; coated tablets should dissolve within 45 minutes. The supplement should have the USP designation on the label.

This means that the supplement meets standards for disintegration (how it breaks into small pieces), dissolution (how it dissolves), strength and purity.

- The product should also have an expiration date on the bottle.

For best results with supplements, keep the following in mind:

- Take supplements with meals. The food will help absorb the vitamins and minerals.
- Take supplements as directed on the bottle. More is not better.
- Avoid taking supplements with coffee, tea or sodas. These beverages could interfere with the absorption of the minerals.
- Take a balanced supplement. The nutrients work together. For example, calcium needs magnesium for best results in the body.
- Trouble swallowing supplements? First place a small amount of liquid in your mouth, then pop in the capsules. Follow with a good gulp of liquid. Some people find liquids that are thicker than water work better for swallowing capsules. Or, you might want to use a liquid with lots of flavour, such as orange or grape juice. If swallowing any tablet or capsule is a crisis, use liquid products or dissolve them in a liquid.

Our bodies need many different nutrients. First and foremost, you need to eat a healthy diet. This would be a diet rich in fruits, vegetables, whole grains, legumes, nuts, seeds and lean protein. Organic foods have frequently been shown to be higher in essential nutrients than conventionally grown foods. Our bodies need more than 50 essential nutrients from vitamins, minerals, proteins, fats and carbohydrates. Eating a variety of foods will help ensure that you will get these nutrients. In addition, foods contain other nutrients which are vital to our health and longevity. For example, plants contain over 12,000 phytonutrients, or biologically active compounds. These phytonutrients help the plant to grow well and ward off diseases and pests. When we eat plants, the benefits of the phytonutrients are passed on to us. Remember, though, that moderate portion sizes of all foods are important to prevent weight gain.

1. BONE-RELATED NUTRIENTS

The main nutrients needed for healthy bones include calcium, phosphorus, magnesium, vitamin D, fluoride and vitamin K.

Calcium:

Besides building bones and teeth, calcium plays a role in nerve transmission, muscle contraction and dilation of blood vessels. Over 99 per cent of the body's calcium is in the bones and teeth. Bone undergoes constant breakdown and rebuilding. In aging adults, the rate of breakdown is greater than that of rebuilding. This leads to bones which become fragile and easily broken. Significant bone loss is known as osteoporosis. People with osteoporosis are at great risk of breaking bones and having the bones in the spine collapse. If folks with MS are inactive, their osteoporosis risk is increased. Corticosteroids dramatically increase the risk of osteoporosis.

Best food sources of calcium are dairy products, tofu, kale, spinach, broccoli, nuts, canned sardines/salmon with bones, molasses, cooked dried peas and beans.

Dietary surveys reveal that most adults do not obtain sufficient calcium from food. Therefore, most adults should consider a calcium supplement of 500 to 1000 mg per day. When choosing a supplement, look for the amount of *elemental* calcium as written on the label. Aim to take calcium carbonate supplements with meals to improve absorption. Other forms of calcium supplements do not need to be taken with food for best absorption. There are many different forms of calcium supplements on the market. They can be liquid, chewable, tablets or capsules. Avoid bone meal and dolomite calcium supplements as they may contain lead. Remember to take your calcium supplement in doses of 500 mg or less for best absorption. When calcium is taken in larger doses, less is absorbed.

RDA: 1000 mg per day for adults aged 19-50
    1200 mg per day for adults over 50
Recommended Supplement:
    500 mg per day for adults aged 19-50
    1000 mg per day for adults over 50
    1500 mg per day for adults at risk of osteoporosis
Upper Level of Tolerable Intake: 2500 mg per day

Phosphorus:
Phosphorus has many roles in the body. Most of the phosphorus in the body is in bones and teeth. Because phosphorus is found widely distributed in foods, deficiency is extremely rare.

RDA: 700 mg per day for adults
Upper Level of Tolerable Intake: 4000 mg per day

Magnesium:
Magnesium is involved in over 300 enzyme systems in the body and is needed for energy production. Over half of the magnesium in our bodies is in the bones. Magnesium intake can be low, especially in people who rely on processed foods. Best sources of magnesium are tofu, legumes, seeds, nuts, whole grains and leafy green vegetables.

RDA: 320 mg per day for women; 420 mg per day for men
Recommended Supplement: 500 mg per day.
Upper Level of Tolerable Intake: 350 mg per day from supplements or medicines.
    Some people take more than this, but must work up slowly and reconsider if diarrhea develops. Toxicity level is: 800-1000 mgs per day.

Vitamin D:
Vitamin D is needed for absorption of calcium and for build-

ing bones and teeth. Food sources of vitamin D are limited. Because of this and because of our northern latitude, Canadians are at risk of vitamin D deficiency.

Best sources of vitamin D include fluid milk, and fortified soy and rice drinks. Butter and eggs contain small amounts of vitamin D. Vitamin D is also added to margarines. The richest natural source of vitamin D is fish, especially fish liver oil. However, do not attempt to meet your vitamin D needs with fish liver oil. Fish liver oil is very high in vitamin A. Taking extra fish liver oil to boost vitamin D intake can result in a toxic intake of vitamin A.

Vitamin D supplements given to people during the winter months have been documented to improve mood. Historically we were programmed to make vitamin D from exposure to sunshine. Now, we live more of an "indoor" existence with limited exposure to the sun. In addition, people use sunscreen and clothing to block the sun's rays on their skin. The consequence is that less vitamin D is produced in the skin. Furthermore, as we age, we produce about one-quarter the vitamin D compared to when we were younger. Dark skinned people are at a greater disadvantage. They require 2 hours or more in the sun to produce the same amount of vitamin D that a light-skinned person produces in 20 minutes.

We feel that the current recommendations for vitamin D are too low. Vitamin D has such a critical role in bone health, in prevention of cancer, in prevention of autoimmune disease and in influencing mood. It is perhaps more of a hormone in its action in the body than a vitamin. There is ample evidence from Vieth's work in Canada and from other researchers that higher levels of vitamin D are required and that levels up to 4000 IU per day is safe.

RDA: 200 IU per day for adults to age 50
　　　400 IU per day for adults 51-70 years
　　　600 IU per day for adults over 70 years
Recommended Supplement:
　　　1000 IU per day for all adults

2000 IU per day for people at risk for osteoporosis

2000 – 4000 IU per day for people with autoimmune disorders or risks of cancer.

Upper Level of Tolerable Intake: 2000 IU per day. Dr. Vieth's research suggests 4,000 IU is safe. If concerned, have your blood concentration measured. See chapter on Vitamin D for details.

Fluroide:

Fluoride helps to stimulate the formation of bones and teeth. It also protects against dental caries.

RDA: 3 mg per day for adult women and 4 mg per day for adult men

2. THE B VITAMINS

The eight B vitamins are: thiamin (B-1), riboflavin (B-2), niacin (B-3), pantothenic acid (B-5), pyridoxine (B-6), cyanocobalamin (B-12), folic acid, and biotin.

Thiamin (B-1):

The main function of thiamin is to help convert carbohydrates into energy. Deficiency of thiamin causes loss of energy, nerve damage and muscular weakness. Chronic alcoholics are at risk of thiamin deficiency. Thiamin also helps to produce acetylcholine, a chemical in the brain which helps with information storage and retrieval. Thiamin activates serotonin, our "feel good" brain chemical. Some studies have shown that a 50 mg thiamin supplement resulted in clearer thinking, more energy and better sleep.

Among the most important food sources of thiamin are whole grains, pork, liver, and cooked dried beans and peas. Many flour and grain products are fortified with thiamin. Thiamin is sensitive to heat and is easily leached out of the food into the cooking water.

RDA: 1.1 mg/day for women; 1.2 mg/day for men

Recommended Supplement: RDA levels are adequate. For improved mood and clearer thinking 50 mg per day is advised.

Upper Level of Tolerable Intake: none (no concerns)

Riboflavin (B-2):

Riboflavin acts with many enzymes to convert food into energy. It is also involved in red blood cell formation, the absorption of iron, the metabolism of B-6 and the production or serotonin and dopamine (neurotransmitters). As with thiamin, recent studies reported that a 50 mg supplement of riboflavin resulted in improved mood and clearer thinking.

Because riboflavin is abundant in the food supply, deficiency is rare. Meats, fish, whole grains, milk products, vegetables and legumes all contain riboflavin. In addition, riboflavin is added to flour and grain products.

RDA: 1.1 mg/day for women; 1.3 mg per day for men
Recommended Supplement: RDA levels are adequate. For improved mood and clearer thinking, 50 mg per day is advised.
Upper Level of Tolerable Intake: none (no concerns)

Niacin (B-3):

Like riboflavin and thiamin, niacin helps convert food into energy. Niacin is also needed for making fatty acids and steroids. Furthermore, niacin is involved in DNA replication and repair. Niacin deficiency is known as pellagra and can occur in chronic alcoholism.

Large doses of niacin are sometimes used to treat high blood cholesterol. These high doses can cause blood vessels to dilate and result in flushing. However, newer niacin formulations are slow release to reduce the flushing effect. High doses of niacin (3-9 gm/day) are toxic to the liver when taken over a prolonged period. Your health care practitioner should monitor this if these amounts are used.

Best food sources are liver, eggs, fish, peanuts, legumes, whole grains, avocadoes, milk, broccoli, pork, potatoes, tomatoes, wheat germ.

RDA: 14 mg/day for women; 16 mg/day for men

Recommended Supplement: RDA levels are adequate.
Upper Level of Tolerable Intake: 35 mg/day.

Pyridoxine (B-6):

B-6 plays an important role in protein metabolism, helping to make amino acids and to break them down for conversion into other compounds or energy. It is needed to synthesize muscle protein, hemoglobin, insulin and antibodies which protect against infection. Vitamin B-6 is essential for the brain to produce serotonin from tryptophan, an amino acid. In addition, B-6 is needed to make DHA, a critical fat needed by the brain. Studies show that people with low DHA levels are more likely to be depressed and that B-6 supplements improve the mood of depressed people.

According to some researchers, almost half of all women consume less than one-half of the RDA for vitamin B-6. In addition, 75% of young women who are restricting calories are deficient in B-6. Other researchers have found that about half of men and women over 50 get the recommended amount of B-6 in their diets. Thus, supplemental B-6 is needed to achieve adequate levels of this vitamin.

Vitamin B-6 is found in a wide variety of foods, including meats, fish, nuts, beans, whole grains and some fruits and vegetables.

RDA: 1.3 mg/day for adults 19-50 years
1.5 mg/day for women over 50; 1.7 mg/day for men over 50
Recommended Supplement: RDA levels are adequate. For improved mood, 50 mg per day are recommended.
Upper Level of Tolerable Intake: 100 mg/day. Large doses of B-6 from supplements have been associated with nerve damage and numbness.

Folate (Folic Acid):

This B vitamin is important for DNA metabolism, cell division and tissue growth. It is also involved in the formation of hemoglobin in red blood cells. Folate is found in green leafy vegetables, peas, oranges, carrots, eggs, bananas, avocado, whole grain, yeast and liver. Folate is easily lost in cooking and processing of foods.

The average intake of folate has been determined to be 242 ug. It is thought that an additional 100 ug would be obtained from fortified foods. Thus, many adults do not get enough folate from food, and a folic acid supplement of 400 ug is recommended. A folic acid supplement is also recommended for all women of child-bearing age, especially in the months before conception. This is because folic acid prevents neural tube birth defects which occur in the first few weeks of pregnancy. Higher levels of folic acid supplementation (5 mg) are recommended in women who have had a miscarriage or who have had a child born with a neural tube defect. Because of the importance of folic acid in preventing birth defects, many foods are now fortified with folic acid.

There is considerable evidence that folic acid may reduce the risk of heart disease and stroke by reducing homocysteine. Homocysteine is a protein in the blood and high levels of this protein have been found in people suffering from heart disease and stroke. Normally, homocysteine is recycled through metabolic reactions with the help of folic acid, vitamin B-12 and vitamin B-6. A level of 1000 ug (1mg) of folic acid is recommended for people with heart disease. It is not known at this time how much supplemental folic acid would be best for prevention of heart disease or stroke. Levels up to 5 mg are currently being researched. However, keep in mind that the Upper Level of Tolerable Intake is 1000 ug. High amounts of folic acid can cover up symptoms of vitamin B-12 deficiency. There is also a concern for people getting too much folate when all sources of folate from food, supplements and food fortification are considered.

The role of folic acid in improving mood has largely been ignored. Over 1/3 of depressed people are deficient in folic acid. Furthermore, it has been shown to improve mood in a study of depressed older patients. The improvement experienced by folate alone was better that that experienced with many antidepressants. Folate does this by helping the body to produce more s-adenosyl methionine or SAMe, a chemical important to mood.

Evidence exists that folate may prevent Alzheimer's disease and Parkinson's disease. Interestingly, high levels of homocysteine have also been reported in people with Alzheimer's and Parkinson's.

RDA: 400 ug per day for adults
Recommended Supplement: 400 ug per day
    1 g per day for people with heart disease and angioplasty
Upper Level of Tolerable Intake: 1000 ug per day (1 mg per day). High levels of folic acid (supplemental) can mask the symptoms of vitamin B-12 deficiency which can have the serious consequence of nerve damage.

Vitamin B-12:
Like folate, B-12 is needed for DNA metabolism. It is also needed for red blood cell formation and maintenance of the nervous system. Animal foods contain B-12; no plant foods contain B-12. However, certain microorganisms, used to ferment foods, can make some B-12. Thus these fermented foods may contain B-12: soy sauce, miso and tempeh.

For certain people, absorption of B-12 can be a problem. In order to absorb B-12, people need a substance called intrinsic factor, which is secreted by the stomach. If a person lacks intrinsic factor, B-12 absorption is not possible. In addition, stomach acid is needed to absorb B-12. In some people, with age, less stomach acid is produced. This can cause malabsorption of B-12, too. Supplemental B-12, either by injection or by capsules is needed to prevent pernicious anemia. If the anemia is severe, it can be followed by nerve damage.

Because many people over the age of 50 have low stomach acid and therefore may not absorb dietary B-12 very well, it is recommended that they should get their B-12 from fortified foods or from supplements. The form of B-12 in supplements is more easily absorbed than the naturally-occurring B-12.

RDA: 2.4 ug per day for adults
Recommended Supplement: 500 ug per day
Upper Level of Tolerable Intake: none (no concerns)

Pantothenic Acid:
This B vitamin is essential for producing and metabolizing fats. It also helps in the formation of hormones and cholesterol. Pantothenic acid is widely distributed in plant and animal foods. Deficiency is extremely rare.

RDA: 5 mg per day
Recommended Supplement: 500 mg per day
Upper Limit of Tolerable Intake: none (no concerns)

Biotin:
Biotin is involved in energy production from food and in the metabolism of fatty acids. Deficiency has only been observed in people eating raw eggs. Raw egg contains a substance which interferes with biotin.

RDA: 39 ug per day for adults
Recommended Supplement: 300 ug per day
Upper Level of Tolerable Intake: none (no concerns)

You will note that there is some flexibility and safety in taking the B vitamins greater than the RDA. If your preferred multivitamin/multimineral does not reach your choice, add a B-complex to this. Often this is much less expensive than searching for an "all-in-one".

3. ADDITIONAL VITAMINS AND TRACE MINERALS

Vitamin A:
Vitamin A is important for normal vision, health of the skin and cells lining the gastrointestinal tract, gene expression,

reproduction, development of the fetus, growth and immune function. Food sources of vitamin A, as retinol, include liver, kidney, butter, cheese, whole milk, fortified low fat and skim milk. Vitamin A, in the form of carotenoids, is found in fruits and vegetables.

Because massive amounts of vitamin A can cause birth defects, an Upper Tolerable Intake Level is established for adults. Vitamin A in high doses can be dangerous because the body stores excessive amounts of this vitamin. This only applies to retinol. The carotenoids, including beta-carotene are non-toxic and are converted to vitamin A in the body only when the body requires more vitamin A.

RDA: 2100 IU per day for women; 2700 IU per day for men
Recommended Supplement: RDA amount
Upper Level of Tolerable Intake: 3000 ug of retinol per day
    (10,000 IU vitamin A)

Vitamin K:
Vitamin K is needed in the production of at least 4 of the 13 proteins involved in blood clotting. It is also important for healthy bones. A deficiency of vitamin K results in slow blood clotting, and in severe cases, bleeding. Vitamin K is found in dark-green leafy vegetables such as Brussels sprouts, lettuce, broccoli, spinach and kale. It is also found in liver, egg yolks and herbal tea and green tea. Some vitamin K is also produced by the beneficial bacteria in our large bowel.

Vitamin K is not sold in supplements in Canada. Vitamin K interacts with the drug Warfarin (Coumadin). Warfarin is used to thin the blood in order to prevent clotting.

RDA: 90 ug per day for women and 120 ug per day for men.
Upper Level of Tolerable Intake: none

Chromium:
A form of chromium, trivalent chromium, helps insulin in regulating glucose and lipid metabolism. Chromium is also

thought to be useful for weight loss because of this insulin response. Food sources of chromium include whole grains, meats, dairy products, brewer's yeast and beer.

RDA: 25 ug per day for women; 35 ug per day for men
Recommended Supplement: 50 ug per day
Upper Level of Tolerable Intake: none

Selenium:
Selenium is a required component of the enzyme glutathione peroxidase, which provides protection from free radicals. Selenium can regenerate vitamin C. In addition, it is involved in the regulation of thyroid hormone. Selenium protects against toxic doses of the heavy metals cadmium, mercury and silver. Selenium deficiency has been linked to cancer and heart disease.

Food sources of selenium include Brazil nuts, dairy products, onions, grains, nuts, chicken, meats, and seafood. The selenium content of foods is dependent on the selenium in the soil where the food is grown. People who live on the west coast of North America, particularly British Columbia, Washington, and Oregon, need to be aware that the soil in these areas is selenium-depleted. Because of this, it may be prudent to include selenium as a supplement.

Recent studies have demonstrated that supplemental selenium at 200 ug/day reduces anxiety, depression and helps to increase energy. It is thought that selenium does this by enhancing dopamine (feel good) levels in the brain.

RDA: 55 ug per day for adults
Recommended Supplement: 200 ug per day
Upper Level of Tolerable Intake: 400 ug per day. The potential for toxicity exists at levels above 800 ug per day. Symptoms of toxicity include hair and nail brittle-ness, gastrointestinal disturbances, skin rash, garlic breath odor, fatigue and irritability.

Copper:
Copper is needed for the synthesis of hemoglobin, the manufacture of collagen, and the maintenance of the myelin sheath that surrounds nerve fibers. It is also necessary for the proper functioning of the heart. Copper is a part of many enzymes involved in making neurotransmitters. Copper is essential for making superoxide dismutase and glutathione peroxidase. Both enzymes quench free radicals, especially those that damage mitochondria, DNA, fats and LDL. Food sources of copper are whole grains, liver, kidney, oysters and nuts. Copper deficiency is rare.

RDA: 900 ug per day for adults
Recommended Supplement: RDA amount
Upper Level of Tolerable Intake: 10,000 ug per day

Iodine:
Iodine is an essential component of the thyroid hormones. Deficiencies of iodine lead to goiter (enlarged thyroid) and inadequate thyroid hormone. Thyroid hormone regulates the body's metabolism. Seafood, saltwater fish and kelp contain iodine. Iodized salt is also available.

RDA: 0.15 mg (150 ug) per day for adults
Upper Level of Tolerable Intake: 1.1 mg (1100 ug) per day

Iron:
About 70% of the iron we absorb from the gut is found in hemoglobin, a protein that releases oxygen to body cells for energy production and gives color to red blood cells. Some iron is also found in muscle cells, other proteins and enzymes. Iron deficiency results in anemia, developmental delays, cognitive impairment, poor pregnancy outcomes and impaired physical performance.

There are many food sources of iron. The iron contained in meat, fish and poultry is better absorbed than the iron found in plant sources. Tea and coffee inhibit iron absorption while vitamin C enhances it.

RDA: 18 mg per day for women of childbearing age; 8 mg
for men
27 mg per day in pregnancy
8 mg per day for postmenopausal women
Recommended Supplement: RDA amounts for women only
Upper Level of Tolerable Intake: 45 mg per day

Manganese:

Manganese is involved in protein and energy metabolism and is essential for normal bone structure. It is also needed for the functioning of the nervous system. Like copper, manganese is involved in producing superoxide dismutase and glutathione peroxidase, which are antioxidants. Manganese is found in legumes and whole grains.

RDA: 1.8 mg per day women; 2.3 mg per day for men
Recommended Supplement: RDA amount
Upper Level of Tolerable Intake: 11 mg per day

Molybdenum:

Molybdenum has been found to be a component of several of the body's enzymes. Molybdenum occurs in meats, grains and legumes.

RDA: 45 ug per day for adults
Recommended Supplement: RDA amount
Upper Level of Tolerable Intake: 2 mg per day

Zinc:

Zinc is an essential component of nearly 100 enzymes. It is the second most abundant trace mineral in the body next to iron. It is required for normal growth and development in children. It is involved in carbohydrate use, in making proteins and in the replication of DNA. Zinc joins copper and manganese in producing superoxide dismutase and glutathione peroxidase. Zinc is found in meats and poultry, oysters, eggs and legumes.

Although zinc deficiency is rare, it can occur. Those at risk include male long-distance runners (zinc is lost in the sweat), alcoholics, and vegetarians.

RDA: 8 mg per day for women; 11 mg per day for men
Recommended Supplement: No more than 30 mg per day
Upper Level of Tolerable Intake: 40 mg per day, based on evidence that high intakes of zinc can impair copper absorption.

4. THE ANTIOXIDANT VITAMINS

Vitamin C:

Vitamin C is a water-soluble antioxidant. In addition, it is a cofactor for enzymes involved in the synthesis of collagen, carnitine and neurotransmitters. Vitamin C also plays a role in wound healing and resistance to infections. Vitamin C provides substantial antioxidant protection of the eye, in white blood cells and in semen. It also protects LDL cholesterol (the bad cholesterol) from being oxidized and contributing to heart disease. Vitamin C has the ability to recycle other antioxidants such as glutathione and vitamin E. Vitamin C has a protective effect against cancers of the oral cavity, larynx, esophagus, lung, stomach, colon, rectum and cervix. In addition, vitamin C is involved in iron absorption, transport and storage.

Vitamin C deficiency is rare in developed countries, but can occur in individuals consuming few fruits and vegetables or in alcoholics. Food sources of vitamin C include vegetables such as broccoli, peppers, potatoes, Brussels sprouts and fruits such as oranges, cranberries, grapefruit, and plums. Exposure of foods to heat and light reduces the vitamin C content. Also, vitamin C can easily be leached out into the cooking water. Prevent vitamin C losses by covering containers of juice and of cut fruits and vegetables.

When a vitamin C supplement is considered, the best form of Vitamin C is esterified C. Esterified C combines minerals like calcium, potassium or zinc with the ascorbic acid.

This makes the supplement non-acidic and more readily absorbed by the body.

RDA: 75 mg per day for women; 90 mg per day for men. Smokers need more vitamin C: women, 110 mg per day; men, 125 mg/day

Recommended Supplement: 500 mg per day

Upper Level of Tolerable Intake: 2 grams per day. High levels of vitamin C cause gastrointestinal upset and diarrhea.

Vitamin E:
Vitamin E is a fat-soluble antioxidant. It protects fats against oxidation. Vitamin E is found in vegetable and seed oils, nuts and seeds, and green and leafy green vegetables. Excellent sources are wheat germ oil, sunflower and safflower oil, peanuts, almonds and soybean, corn and canola oils.

Vitamin E deficiency is rare. Interestingly, the RDA is based only on alpha-tocopherol – the other forms of tocopherol that occur naturally in food are not considered to contribute to vitamin E activity.

Much research has been done on vitamin E to determine its role in disease prevention. A great deal of controversy exists at this time. The bulk of the evidence does not indicate high levels of vitamin E as being beneficial for heart disease. Vitamin E has been shown to be protective against several cancers, including prostate and colon cancer. It is reasonable to suggest that if a vitamin E supplement is taken, it should be in the range of 300-400 IU/day. We suggest a combination of d-alpha, d-gamma and tocotrienol.

RDA: 22 IU (15 mg) per day for adults

Recommended Supplement: 400 IU mixed tocopherols and tocotrienols

Upper Level of Tolerable Intake: 1000 mg per day

The information provided in this chapter only skims the surface of what is known about essential vitamins and minerals and categorizes them according to Bone Related Nutrients, B Vitamins, Additional Vitamins and Trace Minerals and Antioxidant Vitamins. Nutritional science is a young science. Indeed, the first vitamins were only discovered in the early 1900s. Research continues into the roles of nutrients in health and disease. Sometimes the information is contradictory and confusing; other times it is more conclusive. A new area of nutritional research is nutrigenomics. This is the study of the interaction of nutrients with our genetic material. That is, certain nutrients can turn genes on or off, and thus impact on our health and the development of disease. Thus, ongoing research will reveal even more exciting information on how foods and nutrients interact in our bodies to promote healing, health and longevity.

Chapter 10

Antioxidants – Powerful Protection For Today's Lifestyles

Most of us will credit Dr. Linus Pauling for his early approach to antioxidants, especially vitamin C. Although Dr. Pauling was awarded two Nobel prizes, he was decried by most physicians and scientists for promoting what they felt was nutritional quackery. Dr Pauling was a pioneer in nutritional medicine and much of what he promoted has proven to be valid. He believed that nutrition could prevent, help or cure many diseases. He was one of the first scientists that determined free radicals, produced by oxidative stress, could damage all of our body tissues. Let us explore the notion of oxidative stress and the source of these free radicals.

Cells are our body's basic building blocks. We each have some 70 trillion cells making up all our tissues and organs (heart, brain, skin, blood, bones, etc). Our circulating blood delivers the nutrients these cells require and carries away the by-products. Each cell must create its own energy from the food we eat and the oxygen we breathe. This blending or mixing of food and oxygen is called oxidation. A wood burning fire is a superb analogy to the burning of food (fuel) in our bodies. The wood logs represent our food. In order to burn, the fire needs oxygen from the air. The fire releases smoke and carbon dioxide into the air. The heat and light from the fire represent the energy released from the wood.

Just like the fire produces by-products from burning wood for energy, our bodies produce by-products from burning food for energy. When our cells use food for fuel, heat is produced, little packets of energy (ATP, Adenosine Tri-Phosphate) are made and carbon dioxide is given off by our lungs. This compares to the heat and light energy and the carbon dioxide from the wood fire. What do the by-products of smoke and ashes from the fire represent in our bodies? These are the *free radicals* released from the power center in the cell, or mitochondria. Whenever our bodies use oxygen in a process called oxidation, unstable molecules—free radicals—are formed. Indeed, tens of thousands of free radicals are produced naturally in the body every day. A free radical can start a chain reaction in its frenzy to become stable, making other molecules unstable. Thus, anything in the way of free radicals such as proteins, fats or DNA, can be damaged. Free radicals must be stopped. Antioxidants are nature's solution to trapping free radicals and stopping the domino effects of free radical damage.

My next question is: what happens when we exercise and use a lot of energy? We know that we breathe deeper and quicker and that our heart beats faster to supply extra oxygen to our muscle cells. Extra food (calories) is also required. The carbon dioxide is readily breathed out. This burst of oxidation (energy production) produces the extra energy our muscle cells require. As a result of this increased production of energy, a large number of free radicals are released into our muscle cells. These excess free radicals are experienced as physical discomfort in the form of muscle stiffness and soreness over the next 12-36 hours. Thus, exercise is a simple example of "oxidative stress". Irritated muscle cells cry out for their excess free radicals to be "quenched". This is why antioxidants are so important. Antioxidants have the ability to deal with the reactive, damaging free radicals and render them harmless.

If we "supertrain" as an Olympic athlete would need to, then this excess of free radicals must be dealt with by optimal nutrition and nutrition supplements. If not, the heightened free radicals exhaust our cells' antioxidants, including the antioxidant, glutathione, found in our white blood cells. The result is a depressed immune system. Hence we are more vulnerable to infections such as colds or flu viruses, at the time of peak training for competition. Most of us will recall a favorite Olympic athlete who was not performing optimally as a consequence.

Another example of oxidative stress is a partly eaten apple. The exposed fleshy part turns brown over a few hours, due to oxidation. This oxidative stress is precipitated or caused by oxygen contacting the exposed apple. The browning is due to free radical excess. To avoid the browning, we can dip the exposed apple in lemon juice. The vitamin C in this citrus fruit quenches the free radicals, and solves the oxidative stress by supplying an antioxidant.

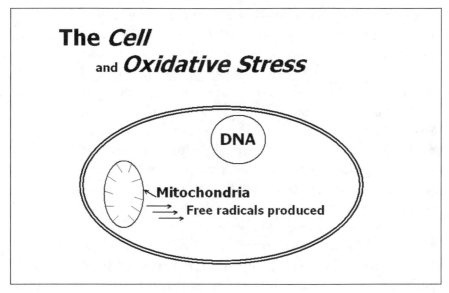

The *Cell* and *Oxidative Stress*

DNA

Mitochondria

Free radicals produced

The Cell and Oxidative Stress: *The outside double lining represents our double layered lipid (fat) cell membrane. DNA is inside the nucleus of the cell. The small egg-shaped oval represents the mitochondria, or power center, which produces energy within the cell. Each cell has many mitochondria to fuel body activity.*

What is it in the cell that is similar to the apple edges turning brown? I will outline this and give three different examples of excess free radicals acting in the cells (i.e. oxidative stress).

Firstly, excess free radicals injure the DNA (deoxyribonucleic acid) which is the blueprint for new cells, DNA and proteins. Injured DNA markedly increases our risk of cancer. Our body produces thousands of new cancer cells daily. Excess free radicals compound or increase this cancer cell production. Certainly those of us with MS do not need another strike against our health to slow us down on our journey to recovery!

Secondly, excess free radicals injure our cell membranes which are made of a double layer of fat (lipid). The cell membrane protects each individual cell and controls what passes into the cell and what the cell releases. If excess free radicals damage the cell membrane, then good and bad components can travel easily in and out of the cell. The cell loses its protective membrane control. Inevitably, the cell is injured and dies early. This is a key step in premature aging. We must heed this warning.

We are actually genetically programmed to live healthy and well to 120-140 years. Changes in hygiene, sanitation and food have improved our chances of this. Unfortunately, the downhill slide of our SAD (Standard American Diet) has shortened our life and increased our chronic and fatal diseases as well. Most of us are dying prematurely in our 60s, 70s and 80s due to degenerative diseases such as heart disease, cancer, stroke and diabetes. Research confirms that degenerative diseases are induced by oxidative stress. We hope to encourage the trend of "whole food junkies". All of us need more "whole foods" such as fruits, vegetables, seeds, nuts and legumes and less processed foods full of salt, sugar and trans fat and devoid of vitamin, minerals and phytonutrients (plant chemicals).

When I was diagnosed with MS in 1996 and then deteriorated for 12 straight months, I felt a poor quality 80 or 90 years of age, at only 43 years of age. I did not expect to see my 50th birthday. Now, I am 51 years "young" and aiming for 100 years! In fact, as I continue to improve physically,

I am starting to hedge my bets. If I feel good at 95, I will move the 100 mark up some! I never thought I would get this much of my life back. You, too, must look after yourself well for many more years, as I do not want to reach 100 and be lonely!

The third part of the cell injured due to free radical excess is the "power center" or mitochondria. Oxidative stress from excess free radicals reduces this power center's ability to produce energy. This is a key factor causing lack of energy in general, and in illnesses such as Chronic Fatigue Syndrome and Fibromyalgia (in Europe it is called Fibromyositis) and probably accounts for the fatigue of MS, Rheumatoid Arthritis, Systemic Lupus Erythematosis and advanced cancers as well.

When I was a General (Family) Practitioner in the early 1980's, I thought I knew what fatigue was. If one of my patients complained of fatigue, I simple sent them for hemoglobin and thyroid lab tests and sometimes, a Monospot to test for infectious mononucleosis. If these were normal, I said, "Good news! You are not tired!" Now, I understand how little I had to offer my "tired" patients. When my MS was severe, I would wake up after 11-13 hours in bed, and still feel "like my arms and legs were nailed down to the bed". This is "fatigue"!

After the above discussion on free radicals and oxidative stress, you can perhaps see how Dr. Linus Pauling was well ahead of his time. Similarly, Hans Selye, and his concepts of emotional, mental and physical stress have been verified. Excessive mental and emotional stress greatly increases free radical production. Pollutants in our air, food and water, cigarette smoke, sunlight, and fatty meals (which also contain trans fats) all increase our production of free radicals. Even medications, chemotherapy and radiation treatments, given in an effort to fight disease, produce free radicals as the body strives to deal with their after-effects. Exercise, especially done excessively, exponentially increases the production of free radicals.

My favorite example when discussing oxidative stress is airplane travel in excess of 4 hours. The triggers of extra free radicals are: reduced oxygen, shared air and viruses and ever-increasing radiation exposure the higher we fly. My recommendation: when you must take an airplane, boost your vitamin C intake with at least a 500 mg supplement or more.

In order to protect our health, now more than ever, we need to reduce the things that produce free radicals and optimize our antioxidant protection. We can never be free of the damaging free radicals, but we can protect ourselves with a blend of antioxidants and then repair oxidative damage with the necessary nutritional building blocks.

Antioxidants are either made in the body or obtained from food or nutritional supplements. Antioxidants made by the body include glutathione, alpha-lipoic acid and Coenzyme Q-10 (CoQ-10). Of all the antioxidants in the body, glutathione is the "master" antioxidant and is discussed more fully in the next chapter. However, most of our antioxidants are obtained from food – another good reason to eat a healthy diet! Vitamin C, vitamin E, plus carotenoids and flavenoids from plants, are found naturally in foods. We can also obtain antioxidants from nutritional supplements.

Alpha lipoic acid is both fat-soluble and water-soluble. This enables lipoic acid to fight free radicals anywhere in the body. Alpha lipoic acid can also work with vitamins C and E and with glutathione to rejuvenate them. This antioxidant has many roles in the body – it prevents LDL (bad cholesterol) oxidation and reduces growth of cancer cells, as well as aiding the immune system. In addition, alpha lipoic acid bonds with toxic metals and helps detoxify the body. For maximum free radical protection, a supplement containing alpha lipoic acid is recommended. Dr. Lester Packer, a world authority on antioxidants recommends a level of 100 mg per day of alpha lipoic acid supplement.

Coenzyme Q-10, which can be made in the body, helps the body produce energy. This is especially important in the high energy areas of the body – the heart, brain, kidneys and liver. As an antioxidant, CoQ-10 works to prevent free radical damage in fatty tissues including the brain and the other high energy areas in the body. Unfortunately, our CoQ-10 production declines with age.

The Japanese have long used CoQ-10 for the treatment of heart disease. It is now known that drugs for lowering cholesterol deplete the body of CoQ-10. Hence people on these drugs, or those with heart disease, would benefit from CoQ-10 supplementation.

CoQ-10 is found in food such as organ meats and salmon. Dr. Packer states that it is nearly impossible to get enough CoQ-10 from diet alone. He recommends a CoQ-10 supplement of 50 mg per day for adults over 40 years of age. For people with heart disease, he recommends an additional 50 mg per day.

Vitamin C, our best known and one of the first discovered antioxidants, is water-soluble. Thus it acts in the blood and within the fluid of the cells. The vitamin C in limes, when fed to sailors, prevented "scurvy". Sailors, after months at sea, and lacking fresh fruits or vegetables, became deficient in vitamin C. In fact, the DRI (Dietary Reference Intake) for Vitamin C (90 mg/day for adult males and 75 mg/day for adult females) is enough to stop scurvy, plus a small safety margin. This does not, however, tell us how much is needed for optimal health, for prevention of chronic disease, or to counteract a sudden burst in extra free radicals. Linus Pauling and many other health and nutrition practitioners, including Denise and I, recommend an intake of vitamin C which is far more than the DRI, and may range from 500 mg per day to 1 to 2 grams per day.

Vitamin C plays an important role to protect the mitochondria in the cell. It can neutralize free radicals before they injure the mitochondria. Vitamin C also boosts the activity of other antioxidants, especially vitamin E. When vitamin E quenches a free radical, it becomes a free radical itself. Vitamin C can then react with the vitamin E to restore it. Scientists have recently discovered that vitamin E can regenerate vitamin C too. Maintaining our levels of vitamins C and E allows continuous regeneration. This is truly a synergistic partnership.

Certainly our second best known antioxidant is Vitamin E. It is a fat-soluble antioxidant and has an important role in protecting the cell membrane from free radical damage. It is also a component of LDL, the "lousy or bad" form of blood cholesterol. Vitamin E has a role in preventing oxidation of LDL and damage to the cells lining blood vessel walls. Both LDL oxidation and blood vessel damage lead to plaque buildup and progression of heart disease. Evidence also exists for vitamin E in protecting the body against aging, arthritis, cancer, cataracts, diabetes and infection. The DRI for Vitamin E is 15 mg per day (22 IU). Again, many health and nutrition practitioners recommend doses of vitamin E in excess of the DRI. However, too much vitamin E can be a problem. Recent studies report that vitamin E beyond 400 IU can be harmful. Therefore, an upper limit of 400 IU is recommended as a supplement. Further individual discussion on vitamins and minerals is in the Vitamins & Minerals Chapter.

An important discovery is that Vitamins C and E, alpha lipoic acid, CoQ-10, and glutathione are network antioxidants. That is, they work together in the body to enhance our health and protect us from disease. These antioxidants work more effectively together and enhance the antioxidant protection. Therefore, they are thought to be especially effective in protecting us from disease and aging.

Another group of antioxidants is the flavenoid group. There are more than 4,000 flavenoids found in plants but the plant foods we commonly eat contain 50 flavenoids. These substances give plants their bright colors and protect the plants from diseases. Plants have been used for thousands of years for their medicinal properties. Research has confirmed that flavenoids are important to our health. Besides being antioxidants, the flavenoids improve memory and concentration, boost the effectiveness of vitamin C, reduce inflammation, improve immune function and protect us from heart disease.

For these reasons, ginkgo biloba, pycnogenol from pine bark, apples, berries, citrus fruits, cruciferous vegetables (broccoli, cauliflower, kale, cabbage and Brussels sprouts), garlic, onions, green leafy vegetables, grapes, wine, soy, tea, walnuts, turmeric, milk thistle and grapeseed extract are rich sources of flavenoids. Everyone is encouraged to include these in his or her diet as often as possible.

Carotenoids are another class of antioxidants obtained from plants. Carotenoids are found in many fruits and vegetables. They are fat-soluble and are absorbed best in the body in the presence of dietary fat. Over 600 carotenoids exist, but only a few are nutritionally significant. Carotenoids are partly responsible for many of the well-documented health benefits of diets rich in fruits and vegetables.

Carotenoids have many health benefits. Because they protect DNA from free radical damage, they play a role in cancer prevention. For example, diets high in lycopene and high blood levels of lycopene are associated with decreased prostate cancer risk. Beta-carotene and lycopene protect the skin from ultraviolet radiation damage. Lutein works to prevent cataracts and macular degeneration. Lutein and lycopene protect against cardiovascular diseases. At this time, no RDA has been established for carotenoids.

No one antioxidant can protect the body from all the free radicals. Because there are such a wide variety of antioxidants in our food supply, aim to eat a variety of different plant foods every day. Aim for *at least* 5 servings of fruits *and* vegetables daily. Eight to 10 servings would be better! (The average North American only eats 2-3 servings of fruits and vegetables daily. A serving is a one-half cup portion of fruit, vegetable or juice.) In fact, in 2005, the United States government revised the Dietary Guidelines for Americans to include *more* Fruits and Vegetables. Americans are now encouraged to eat 2 cups of fruits per day and 2 and one-half cups of vegetables. This amount is based on a 2000 calorie diet for adults and reflects 4 servings of fruit and 5 servings of vegetables. Canadians should take note: Health Canada is currently reviewing Canada's Food Guide and no doubt, recommendations will be forthcoming that also encourage more fruits and vegetables.

Eating lots of fruits and vegetables, especially brightly

coloured ones, will provide your body with many different antioxidants. The overall benefits will be greater than if you only have a few antioxidants. Select antioxidant supplements to complement your intake of antioxidants from foods. Science cannot yet tell us what level of antioxidant protection we need individually. However, there is overwhelming evidence for the role of antioxidants in promoting health, preventing chronic diseases, and treating illness.

In recognition of the health benefits of antioxidants, many products now appear on store shelves. Capsules with dried fruit and vegetable mixtures, plant-based powders, fruit and vegetable bars, juices and many other plant-based supplements are now available. As with all products, consumer beware. Quality varies, as do components. Many consumers are bewildered by the choices. Do read labels and check out the proportions of the various ingredients. Read promotional materials carefully. Ask the same questions that you would ask when choosing vitamin/mineral supplements. You can review these in the previous chapter on vitamins and minerals.

Our world economy also gives us access to foods not normally found in North America. Some of these foods have tremendous potential for our health. In particular, two new juices are worthy of mention. The first juice is a product made with mangosteen and the second juice combines four unusual and highly nutritious juices.

Mangosteen, grown in Southeast Asia, has been a traditional medicine for treatment of skin infections and wounds for years. The active compounds in the mangosteen are called xanthones. Xanthones have been shown to be antibacterial, anti-inflammatory, and antifungal. Scientific studies indicate that mangosteen may help depression, pain, inflammation and cancer. The mangosteen also provides antioxidant protection. For the greatest benefits from mangosteen, the whole fruit, including the outer covering, or pericarp, should be included with the juice.

The second juice is a mixture of gac juice, Chinese lycium, Siberian pineapple and cili fruit. Gac juice contains carotenoids bound to fatty acids. These carotenoids, called lipocarotenes, enhance the absorption of antioxidants and nutrients. Gac is especially rich in lycopene, betacarotene and vitamin E. It has ten times more betacarotene than carrots and 70% more lycopene than tomatoes.

Siberian pineapple, also known as sea buckthorn, is native to Siberia and the Himalayas. It has a long history of use for rejuvenation and as a blood purifier. Siberian pineapple is high in vitamins A, C and E, B vitamins and minerals. Over 110 studies support its use for heart disease, eye health, periodontal health, immune function and liver function.

Chinese lycium has been used in Traditional Chinese Medicine for over 2000 years. It is known for its antioxidant effects and antiaging effects. This fruit contains forty times more zeaxanthin than corn. Zeaxanthin is a carotenoid that is important for eye health (macular degeneration).

The fourth fruit in the juice mixture is cili fruit from China. This fruit has sixty times more vitamin C than oranges. It also contains polyphenols, which belong in the antioxidant flavenoid family.

The combination of these four impressive fruits into a single beverage results in a nutrient-rich juice. The juice is backed by a significant amount of research. Studies show that this super fruit juice provides antioxidant protection and cellular rejuvenation as well as supporting healthy immune function.

Nature provides us with an exciting array of plants. Science will continue to reveal the different components in plants and how they contribute to our health. Even if we do not yet understand how these phytonutrients, or plant chemicals, work in our bodies, one thing we know for sure. We know that we should eat plenty of fruits and vegetables, especially the brightly colored ones. They are our passports to vibrant health.

As humans looking for evidence of proof, we like to measure things and have objective information. This is especially true as it applies to our health. We measure our height, weight, blood pressure, cholesterol and blood sugar in order to evaluate our health. We might question our iron status, our B-12 status or our vitamin D status. People often wonder too, if they are getting enough vitamins and minerals. Levels of these can be obtained from blood samples. However, these are inconvenient and typically quite expensive.

In addition, some measurements reflect a brief window in time and hence, are of little use. A good example would be vitamin C, which is water-soluble and only lasts several hours. Similarly, vitamin E lasts only several days, despite being fat-soluble. Measurement of other antioxidants like lycopene and other carotenoids is not commonly done and therefore difficult to access. Given the health benefits of antioxidants, how can they be measured reliably, quickly and with minimal expense? Surely, it is to everyone's benefit to know how well their body is protected by antioxidants.

Fortunately, there is a new option recently on the market in North America and now in many other countries in the world. Research by a physicist, Dr. Werner Gellerman at the University of Utah, has focused on reading the carotenoid antioxidants, lutein and zeaxanthin at the back of the eye (retina). This determination could have considerable impact on preventing macular degeneration – the most common cause of blindness. The equipment developed for this purpose was called a biophotonic scanner.

Serendipity expanded this research when a graduate student noticed that this biophotonic scanner did a "reading" from the palm of her hand. Extensive testing revealed the scanner's ability to read 18 different carotenoids from the fat pad of the palm between the little finger and the wrist. Comparisons with blood testing at the same time validated the measurement of this subset of antioxidants. Similarly, there is reasonable inference of vitmian C and vitamin E adequacy. The company, based in Salt Lake City, continues to pay royalties to the University of Utah on this innovative antioxidant testing technique.

Now, for the first time ever, individuals can determine their antioxidant protection with the biophotonic scanner. The scan is a quick, non-invasive and accurate way to determine *skin carotenoid score,* or SCS. More and more people are understanding the link between antioxidant status and health. The SCS score can be obtained every month or two. Thus a person can determine if he/she is improving or losing the free radical battle with respect to lifestyle and to the antioxidants ingested from food and supplements. Low scores underscore the need to pay more attention to diet or to quality and quantity of supplements. Low scores also mean that one should analyze lifestyle and environment to determine any factors that may contribute to oxidative stress. Factors that contribute to oxidative stress and exposure to free radicals include excess body fat, tobacco smoke, stress, sunlight, pollution and environmental toxins.

Thus, our bodies are subjected to free radicals that are produced internally and those that result from exposure to our external environment — our air, water and food. The biophotonic scanner heralds a new era in nutrition. Now we can optimize our dietary intake, including supplements, to our surroundings, or optimize our personal stress, air, water, food and environment. We are now in "control" of our well-being, and we truly "are what we swallow or eat".

Such objective evidence can now help determine our individuality regarding our 1) genetic inheritance, 2) diet, 3) supplement quality and 4) personal stress. Such knowledge can only enhance our health. Don't you wonder what your SCS score is? For further information on antioxidants and the biophotonic scanner, see Resources at the end of this book.

Chapter 11

Glutathione

Glutathione (glu the tie on), abbreviated as GSH, is the body's master antioxidant and is found in every body cell. It is a small protein, which is produced naturally in the body from three amino acids (glycine, glutamine, and cysteine). GSH is essential to life – without it, we die. The scientific literature has over 50,000 articles discussing GSH and its importance to health. Indeed, this tiny protein is known as the body's essential health AID for its **A**ntioxidant protection, **I**mmune system modulation and its ability to **D**etoxify the body.

GSH is a new concept. Most people are not aware of its role in health and most health professionals have only a vague idea of its importance. Soon, GSH will become common knowledge, much as cholesterol and blood sugar are today. All health care practitioners, including physicians, will want to know the glutathione levels of their patients. Why will this happen? GSH levels are an indicator of health and of how long a person will live.

Currently, GSH measurement is done by a blood sample and costs approximately $50 - $120 CDN or $40 - $100 USD. Measurement of GSH reflects GSH concentration in the body over several weeks. The red blood cells are frozen, to breakdown the cell membrane and hence the measurement of GSH reflects the its concentration inside the cell or, its cytoplasmic concentration.

The importance of GSH was reflected in a 2004 edition

of the New England Journal of Medicine. Glutathione peroxidase (an enzyme in the glutathione building pathway) was touted as being the best predictor of a heart attack – surpassing C-reactive protein (CRP). (Elevated levels of CRP are found in people with heart disease). GSH and glutathione peroxidase are directly related. Neither will be produced in excess in the body, as each has a major protective feedback loop to prevent this. In the future, GSH measurement will supercede cholesterol, C-reactive protein, the ESR (Erythrocyte Sedimentation Rate) and probably glutathione peroxidase.

I initially knew GSH as the number one body component for detoxifying or removing drugs used in medicine or intravenous anesthesiology. Despite knowing this, I had no idea how I could potentially raise my personal GSH. This changed for me in late 2001.

I had just completed a seminar on "Nutrition for Mood & Mind", in our local city of Duncan, British Columbia, Canada. Following the question period, a fellow came up, thanked me for the lecture, and asked if I had ever heard of GSH. I replied "yes", to this, because of my teaching and academic experience in anesthesiology. However, I was unable to answer how one could do this with food.

In fact, we are relatively unable to raise our body's intra-cellular GSH with regular food, GSH capsules, or even n-acetyl-cysteine (NAC) by mouth. Considerable GSH is present in many fruits, vegetables and meats. Being a protein, GSH is routinely digested into its three amino acids: glycine, glutamine and cysteine. Cysteine, alone in the gut after GSH digestion, is a sulfur-containing amino acid and is treated as a free radical. It is almost immediately oxidized to a charged molecule. Very little of this single, charged, cysteine amino acid is able to pass through the gut lining into our bloodstream. Similarly, very little of this small amount of cysteine is able to enter the cells throughout the body.

NAC, if given by mouth, is only slightly more successful in raising general body cell's GSH. Only 6-10% is absorbed through the gut and very little is taken up into the body cells. Almost zero NAC is able to cross the blood brain barrier. This is indeed unfortunate, as many brain illnesses are worsened due to the lack of glutathione inside brain cells – i.e. neurons and astrocytes (glial cells).

What would we find if we measured blood GSH in those people with brain illnesses, particularly MS? Once diagnosed with either MS or Parkinson's, both neurodegenerative diseases, the body's cellular GSH is only 5% of what it should be. Similarly, limited brain GSH is key in the development of either ALS (Amylotrophic Lateral Sclerosis) or Alzheimer's. The severity of injury from stroke, brain injury or brain trauma is greatly affected by brain cell GSH as well.

The story of the best way to raise GSH in our body's cells is entertaining, exciting and all-Canadian. It began with the immigration from Italy of an Italian-trained surgeon, Dr. Gustav Bounous. Dr. Bounous became a lab-based researcher, first in Indiana, then in Sherbrooke, Quebec, Canada and finally settled in Montreal, Quebec, Canada, at McGill University.

In 1967, Dr. Bounous and his associate received a Gold Medal from the Royal College of Physicians and Surgeons of Canada for groundbreaking research in human nutrition. His discovery led to his being funded by the Medical Research Council of Canada. Dr. Bounous was the researcher who developed the "elemental" diet of simple amino acids, fatty acids and sugars that was tolerated by patients recovering after a major surgery or in intensive care. Dr. Bounous continued his quest for the optimal protein diet to recover from any major body stress.

One day, a box of pure whey protein arrived on his desk from a Swiss dairy company, with a cheque attached. The dairy company hoped Dr. Bounous could determine a medical or economic use for their whey. Whey was a very common by-product of European cheese production. Dr. Bounous gave this whey protein to his laboratory mice and was astounded to find they lived 30 to 50% longer than when they consumed other equivalent protein diets.

Dr. Bounous then began working on the method or mechanism of why this whey protein isolate was so unique. However, about this time, his lab experiments quit working. He was still receiving the whey protein from the same company in Europe, sent by the same courier. For the next 30 months, he was unable to reproduce the previous results of the very exciting 30-50% life extension in mice fed the protein.

Then, serendipity intervened. While watching television one evening, Dr. Bounous learned that 30 months previously, a salmonella outbreak had occurred in Europe. Subsequent to this, the European health authorities had raised the minimum pasteurization temperature by 3^0C. Dr. Bounous felt that the slight rise in pasteurization temperature might be responsible for the lack of results. He could barely wait to resume his research from a North American whey protein isolate, which might enable him to restart his success with longevity. Indeed, it worked!

About this time, Dr. Bounous was joined in his research by a world class U.K. Immunologist, Dr. Patricia Kongshavn. These two researchers combined their respective talents and energies to unlock the secrets of this whey protein isolate and how it worked in our bodies.

They determined that any fresh or carefully pasteurized source of mammalian whey isolate could have profound benefit. For those intuitive among us, this would fit with our premise that fresh breast milk is the optimal food for human babies.

Drs. Bounous and Kongshavn went on to find that 10 grams (0.3 ounce) of white powder from this whey protein isolate could be obtained from one liter (U.S. quart) of human breast milk. The process used to obtain the whey protein isolate was patented (US Patent # 5,451,412). These researchers demonstrated that 4-5 liters or 4-5 quarts of cow's milk was needed to produce 10 grams (0.3 ounce) of the same whey protein isolate. This disparity is due to human breast milk being 80% whey protein and 20% casein (cheese) protein; meanwhile, cow's (sheep's or goat's, etc) milk is 20%

whey and 80% casein. The milk is pasteurized at the lowest possible temperature and then micro-filtered through a ceramic unit to further eliminate any bacteria.

All milk is obtained from strictly vegetarian cows, including testing to eliminate milk containing antibiotics or hormones to enhance milk production. The whey is the most desired product in this instance. Casein is removed and sold as a by-product to a cheese company. Similarly, all the fat (fatty acids) are removed and almost all the lactose. This permits most of us to take this specialized whey protein isolate, a white powder, without lactase enzymes. However, the extremely lactose sensitive, my sister is one, should take lactase alone, or with a plant digestive enzyme containing lactase. For more on enzymes, see Chapter 7 on food sensitivity and MS.

What is so special about this patented whey protein? The most unique component is "bonded cysteine" maintained within it. This bonded cysteine consists of two cysteine amino acids (all of which contain sulfur) held together by a "gentle" but all important disulfide bond.

What is a disulphide bond and how do each of us frequently experience the same thing in our own hair? Each hair is a strand of protein. Freshly washed hair tends to flatten after 2 or 3 days. This "flat" hair results from many, many disulfide bonds or bridges forming between strands of hair. These multiple bridges routinely form in unwashed hair after 2-3 days. How do we "break" most of these bridges? We apply water, shampoo, rinse with water and towel dry. Now our hair is fluffy again. This example illustrates how easy it is to "break" this gentle disulfide bond.

This "bonded cysteine", uniquely present in all fresh mammalian milk, has several special properties. Firstly, it is protected from digestion in the gut by our own digestive enzymes, pepsin and trypsin. Secondly, this bonded cysteine is a neutral or uncharged molecule and readily passes through the gut lining into our bloodstream. The heart circulates this blood, rich in bonded cysteine, to all body tissues including the brain. Yes, this bonded cysteine also crosses the blood brain barrier. Once this uncharged particle is in the fluid surrounding our cells it readily enters all of our cells. The bonded cysteine supplies two cysteine molecules which are each able to combine with glycine and glutamine to form GSH.

Drs. Bounous and Kongshavn and other researchers have now learned that the rate limiting raw material for the production of intracellular GSH is cysteine. Each cell's own enzymes readily cleave the "bonded cysteine's" disulfide bond and this problem is now solved.

In addition, the cell will never make more GSH than it needs due to the protective and carefully regulated feedback loop of GSH production. We now know GSH is also an important way for the body to store this critical cysteine amino acid. In fact, Dr. Wulf Dröge, in the journal FASEB in 2001, described how the cysteine molecule is the critical controller of protein energy malnutrition, and our healing process!

This is also a very significant piece of the puzzle in healing issues for the person with MS and other neurodegenerative illnesses. Certainly, boosting one's intake of bonded cysteine with four packets (10 gms each) daily, of this "legal white powder" will heal almost any bed sore or "pressure ulcer" within 30-90 days, when added to regular wound care techniques.

The skin is the "mirror" of the body's well being. Therefore, if the skin wound can heal, so will other tissues as well. This includes muscle cells and even brain cells. Similarly, the body always heals with inflammation (remember redness, swelling, heat & pain or loss of function) and optimal GSH also fine-tunes or minimizes inflammation. Subsequently, swelling (heat, redness & pain too) is less, healing is faster and scar formation is also minimized. This sounds very good to me as an MS sufferer! This means less acute symptoms of MS, secondary to the swelling of inflammation, with our most obvious being a change in vision. In addition, it negates or reduces a major indication for a "pulse" of intravenous cortiscosteroids, with their many unhappy side effects.

GSH, inside the body, has three key functions as previously mentioned. The acronym AID describes this quite well – A is for Antioxidant, I is for Immune system modulation or fine-tuning and D is for Detoxification (see Chapter 8). The previous chapter on antioxidants introduced you to oxidative stress, free radicals and many of our exogenous or "outside the body" antioxidants. GSH is our number one, or master antioxidant and must be made inside the cell, as just discussed.

If adequate GSH can be made inside the cell it can minimize excess free-radical injury to, 1) the DNA, and hence reduces cancer, 2) the cell membrane, prolonging cell life and therefore anti-aging, and 3) the power center or mitochondria of the cell, which enhances energy production within the cell. It is this last feature that has enabled me to recover most of my energy and helped give me much of my life back. Today's "energy illnesses" such as chronic fatigue syndrome, fibromyalgia and probably also the fatigue of MS, rheumatoid arthritis, lupus and most debilitating illnesses can be improved by raising the GSH inside the cells.

It is now understood that adequate or optimal GSH inside the cells can "recycle" or rejuvenate both vitamin C and E. Hence, I currently supplement with only 300 units of vitamin E and 500 mgs of vitamin C daily. Previously, I had to "guess" how much I needed for optimal quenching of free radicals. This also optimizes the body's use of other antioxidants such as coenzyme Q-10, alpha lipoic acid and others.

Optimal function of the immune system, or white blood cells, is also dependent on the GSH inside these cells. We now realize that the GSH can fall to one half of optimal in just four to five hours. So, if we can optimize this GSH inside our white blood cells, several key changes occur. Our white blood cells act in two major groups – B-cells and T-cells.

B-cells, or humoral white blood cells, are responsible for making our antibody proteins. These attack and combine with foreign proteins, or body proteins the body thinks are foreign. This is the basis of most of our allergic response

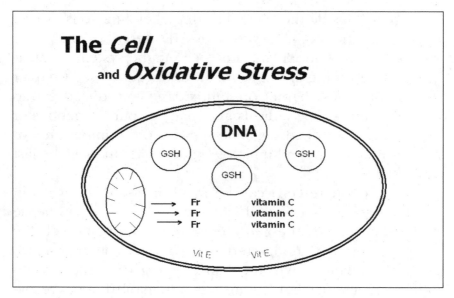

Although not drawn to scale, the above diagram depicts the GSH molecules which are primarily inside the cell. Without enough GSH in the cell, each vitamin C or E molecule must combine with a free radical and take it all the way out of the body. Whenever there is adequate GSH in the cell then both vitamin C or E molecules can combine with a free radical, drop the free radical off at the GSH, go and get another, and so on. Now, the cells are able to recycle their vitamin C and E, so less guesswork as to how much to supplement vitamin C and E is solved. Also, a GSH molecule can combine with a heavy metal (mercury or lead) and remove that toxin from the body. GSH does similar clearing of drugs once they have acted on the cell receptors and done their job.

(such as hay fever and even asthma) and our autoimmune diseases such as MS, rheumatoid arthritis, lupus, inflammatory bowel diseases, type-1 juvenile onset diabetes, and so on.

T-cells are primarily responsible for cell-mediated immunity within our body. This is the white blood cell function of attacking bacteria, viruses, fungi, cancer cells and even the antigen-antibody complexes created by the humoral or B-cells. It is now understood that this shift towards cell-mediated immunity from humoral or antigen-antibody immunity reduces not only our hypersensitivity or hyperactive allergic response but also the severity of our autoimmune diseases.

For those of us with a chronic illness such as MS, this also permits fewer bacterial infections such as bladder infections and sinusitis. Similarly, the raised GSH in the brain cells (neurons, astrocytes), and in cells surrounding a neuron being attacked by our own white blood cells, will minimize the free radicals produced, thereby injuring a small area rather than a large area. I'll try to explain how this enhanced GSH in our white blood cells modulates their function, rather than simply boosts it.

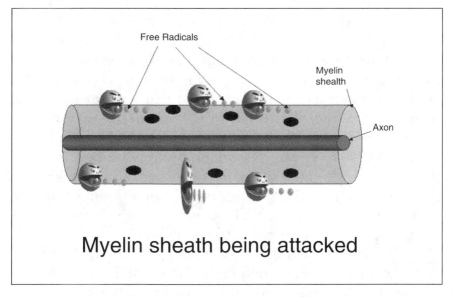

Myelin sheath being attacked

The dark central core represents the nerve's axon. The shaded area around it represents the myelin sheath. The black ovals, seven of them, represent our own white blood cells attacking the myelin. The tiny, shaded circles represent free radicals given off. The "pac men" represent the surrounding astrocytes, neurons and oligodendrocytes, which become injured as the free radicals get to them.

"Boosting" the immune system per say, will frighten many of us lay people, and even some family physicians. Heretofore, their understanding of autoimmune illness was an overactive immune system. For example, once diagnosed with MS, my personal physician suggested I stay away from echinacea. Her anxiety was based on the premise that because echinacea boosted my immune system, it could worsen my MS. Similarly, I have learned some physicians have pitched in the garbage their MS patients' GSH building blocks, whey protein isolate, for the same reason. Happily, this is not a problem, as the "simple" boost is more correctly understood as a modulation, fine-tuning or even optimization of our white blood cell function. Therefore, it helps relieve rather than aggravate the autoimmune illness, MS. I feel raising my GSH is one of the biggest pieces (30%) of my own MS recovery puzzle. It could have a similar benefit in your MS journey.

What did I do when I first learned about building up my GSH with these 10 gm (0.3 oz) packets of the whey protein isolate? I started carefully, and cheaply, of course! This meant one packet per day, mixed in fruit juice, water, milk, yogurt or applesauce. In addition, I learned **not to** heat it (especially above 140°F or 55°C) or **not to** mix it in a blender, as this might break this very important bridge of "bonded cysteine". My new friend Mike, who had initiated this idea for me, also mixed my first packet at my kitchen table! Mike stirred the powder in a small amount of orange juice with a fork. He then added a little more orange juice. I drank the mixture saying it tasted pretty decent.

I then proceeded to try and mix my own, daily for two days. Luckily, Mike phoned back 2 days later asking how it was going. "It's not!" I replied. Mixing the powder was a real hassle so I had given up. Plan B, and then Plan C was presented. Plan B, or low tech, consisted of a shaker cup, not unlike one used to start making a gravy paste. Plan C, or "hi-tech", consisted of a tiny, hand-held mixer, held below the liquid level of the powder (or else it goes everywhere, quickly!) Each of these methods works quite adequately, but a spoon helps consume the bubbled, froth or lumps. I have also since discovered that a bit of fat from oil or cream can help minimize lumps.

Now that a safe, effective means exists for raising GSH in the body, I would recommend that anyone with a chronic illness try this specialized whey protein isolate. It may take 2 packages, or more, over a 6-month period to experience any benefit. The health benefits far outweigh the difficulty mixing and the expense of buying this "white powder".

Before ending the discussion on this GSH enhancing, or key building block whey protein isolate, I want to comment on its safety. It is a food. The U.S. government has granted is GRAS status, i.e. generally regarded as safe. People are sensitive or allergic to this "humanized" milk protein only one in a hundred thousand. Also, for the last five years it has been listed as a dietary supplement for cancer and AIDS in the PDR (Physician's Desk Reference) and the Pharmacists Red Book – both are key standard texts in the U.S.A. Refer to **www.emu.ca** for links for more information.

Chapter 12

Vitamin D- More Than Sunshine

One of the most under-rated and least-understood nutrients is vitamin D, the "sunshine vitamin". For years, vitamin D has only been associated with strong bones and teeth. However over the past ten years, some fascinating information regarding the many roles of vitamin D has surfaced. Most health professionals, including dietitians and physicians, either have not heard this information, or if they have, they have greeted it with a great deal of skepticism. Denise and I strongly believe that vitamin D is one of the key pieces of the "MS Recovery Puzzle". We give credit to those brave and wise scientists who have started the vitamin D ball rolling. It is a message that everyone needs to pay attention to. But first, here is some background information.

A comprehensive review called, "Sunlight Robbery", by Oliver Gillie, describes the link between vitamin D and evolution, and the strong association between inadequate vitamin D and chronic illness. As evidence, he cites over 200 scientific documents.

Humans have always needed vitamin D and this need was demonstrated as changing skin colour as our ancestors moved away from the equator and to the north and to the south. At the equator, the dark-skinned people had ample sunshine year-round to make vitamin D in their skin. As they moved from the equator, they received adequate sunlight on bare skin for only part of the year. Consequently, people developed lighter skin to allow for greater vitamin D production during the time that sunshine was effective. Keep in mind that given the same sunlight exposure, pale skin makes vitamin D six times faster than dark skin. Vitamin D is linked to fertility, thus it was the paler-skinned children who were able to grow and be healthy.

We now know that in mid-summer at the 49th parallel (along the USA-Canada border) a "white-skinned" person with short sleeves and no hat makes 10,000 units of vitamin D in 20 minutes. Similarly, a dark-brown or black-skinned person requires 40-60 minutes to make the same amount of vitamin D. You may already be ahead of me in realizing that Northern Europeans (the "hotbed" of MS) such as Scandinavians in Norway, Sweden, Denmark and Finland, and Celts in Ireland and Scotland, are often very fair skinned. This change would have occurred relatively quickly, over thousands of years, due to the impact of vitamin D concentration on fertility. This was truly, "the survival of the fittest."

Vitamin D is fat-soluble. Hence, the fat in the body can maintain it for up to two months, but very little beyond this. This explains why Embry, Snowdon and Vieth in the annals of Neurology, August 2000, note that MS symptoms and MS lesions or changes on MRI in people in Germany with MS, have seasonal fluctuations. They noted that within two months of the end of their summer (mid or late September) that the MS patients were having relapses. Van de Mei and colleagues (2001) also demonstrated that MS prevalence in various regions in Australia was dependent on the ultraviolet radiation. They found a close association between theoretical prevalence predicted from ultraviolet radiation levels (sunshine) and actual MS prevalence.

Work by Vieth in Canada has further enhanced our knowledge of vitamin D and its safety. In the American Journal of Clinical Nutrition (1999), he determined that Canadians in their 50's and 60's could readily and safely take 4,000 IU of vitamin D-3 (cholecalciterol) daily for six months. Happily, none of their vitamin D-3 measurements exceeded mid-range. Similarly, I have taken 4,000 IU of vitamin D-3 daily for six years and my vitamin D-3 measures 99, normal range being 30-150 nmol/liter. 4000 IUs of vitamin D, daily, sounds less ominous if translated to milligrams where it is 0.1 mgs daily. People with gut absorption concerns, especially fat, may need to take more. I have a woman colleague, who, after taking 4,000 units per day for 5 years, found her vitamin D-3 only measured 30.

Current estimates for optimal blood levels of vitamin D-3 to minimize MS symptoms, are 90-110 nmol/l. In four studies, 10,000 IU per day (250 micrograms) orally of vitamin D-3 is equivalent to full skin body exposure to sunlight for 25-30 minutes. An early study by Stamp confirmed vitamin D-3 supplementation was as effective as sun exposure. Further research shows oral vitamin D-3 (a by-product of sheep's wool or pigskin source), more effective than vitamin D2 (yeast source). Therefore, I recommend 4,000 IU of vitamin D-3 minimum if you have an autoimmune illness such as MS. This 4,000 IU is equal to 0.1 mgs, or 100 micrograms and will cost you about 5 cents per day. I take this year-round, despite sun exposure in our Canadian four-month summer window.

Vitamin D is now known to reduce the risk of at least 16 cancers including bowel, prostate, breast and ovarian cancers. There is also strong evidence for vitamin D's role in preventing Type 1 diabetes and, reduced levels of vitamin D induce insulin resistance which is a risk for Type 2 diabetes. Low levels of vitamin D have also been linked to obesity, high blood pressure, muscle weakness in the elderly, depression, inflammatory bowel disease, rheumatoid arthritis and heart failure. In addition, vitamin D has a beneficial effect on our immune system in regards to healing infections, particularly tuberculosis and other autoimmune illnesses such as psoriasis.

Janet Raloff wrote a two-part series in **www.science-news.org** in 2004, Part I and II "Vitamin D, What Is Enough?" Her summary of the story of vitamin D would at first appear simple. "Take in enough sun, or drink enough fortified milk to get the recommended daily amount, and you'll have strong bones. Take a supplement if you want insurance. But recent studies from around the world have revealed that sunshine's vitamin role in health, is far more complex. More than just protecting bone, vitamin D is proving to preserve muscle strength and to give some protection against deadly diseases including multiple sclerosis (MS), diabetes, and even cancer."

This means that vitamin D is more like a hormone than a vitamin. Bone-metabolism specialist, Robert P. Heaney, states vitamin D is a misnomer. "A vitamin is an essential food constituent that the body can't make." He expands by explaining that we make vitamin D in our skin from a cholesterol-like precursor. Our body can generate 10,000 to 12,000 units, (250 to 300 micrograms) of vitamin D in 30 minutes of summer sunshine. And yet, most people in the USA get well below the recommended 200 to 600 IU per day especially in winter. We Canadians and northern Europeans are particularly in need of vitamin D supplementation because of the lack of effective sunshine for vitamin D production from October to April. We know from Canadian studies of blood vitamin D levels, that adults have a blood level below 40 in winter months. This is far too low to reap the health benefits seen with higher blood levels of vitamin D. When we heed dermatologists' warning about preventing skin cancer by limiting sun exposure and using sunscreen, we also reduce our vitamin D production. At present, there is a visible lawsuit proceeding, involving an early advocate of increased vitamin D. In Boston, Dr. M.F. Holick is suing to get his academic position back. It was "stripped" from him because of his vitamin D position being too far outside the opinion of the major American scientific community. I am supporting Holick on this one!

Bischoff-Ferrari, now at Harvard, measured vitamin D blood concentrations in elderly men and women. Individuals with higher readings also had greater thigh strength. Bischoff-Ferrari then launched an intervention trial with 122 women in their mid-80's. Everyone received 1,200 mgs of calcium per day, and half received 800 IU of vitamin D.

After three months, each woman was tested for leg strength and how easily she could get up from a chair, walk around an object and sit back down. Not only did the vitamin D supplemented women perform dramatically better, but they also sustained only half as many falls. Falls of course are a leading cause of fracture and disability and are believed to cost $20 billion U.S. each year in medical bills.

You can see clearly from the above study that vitamin D supplementation is more than just "slowing down" or "reversing" osteoporosis. It is no longer just enough to have the long recommended DRI, because this amount is only enough to prevent rickets. Rickets, (bowed legs in children), is actually on the increase in Canada and the United Kingdom. Dark skinned children are especially at risk, as they require more time in the sunshine to make the same amount of vitamin D. In addition, careful studies of pregnancy and time of year of delivery, reveal that those born in spring, are more at risk of MS because the pregnant moms tend to have much less vitamin D in winter months. Better protection exists for babies born in late autumn due to more vitamin D. Some nutrition experts are suggesting vitamin D supplementation (I suggest at least 1,000 IU, though I like 2,000 IUs better) is as important in pregnancy as folic acid. Of course, the newborn child should be on a vitamin supplement containing vitamin D immediately. We know that 1,000 IU of vitamin D in a one-year old infant and onwards, much reduces that child's risk of Type 1 diabetes, MS, rheumatoid arthritis, and childhood cancers. In addition, there is considerable increased risk of MS in my own children, due to the fact that myself and a sister have both been diagnosed with MS. If only one parent, it is 2-3% risk, but it more than doubles if a parent's sibling also has MS. 4000 IU, 100 micrograms, of vitamin D is very inexpensive, safe and serves as a valuable health insurance.

Osteoporosis prevention has inclined many calcium product manufacturers to include vitamin D in the calcium supplement. However this is only a small, very modest amount of vitamin D. Often this is 200 IU per 500 MG calcium. The vitamin D helps improve absorption of calcium from the gut from 20-30% up to 80%. Calcium is best absorbed with food and, ideally, only 500 mg of elemental calcium should be taken at one time. Larger doses of calcium are not as effectively absorbed.

Besides limited amounts of sunshine to produce adequate vitamin D in the body, we also have a problem in getting enough vitamin D from food. Vitamin D sources include fish liver oils, fish like salmon, mackerel and sardines and eggs. Small Amounts of vitamin D are found in pork and beef liver and butter. To prevent rickets, Health Canada realized years ago that supplemental vitamin D was needed. This led to vitamin fortification of fluid milk and of margarine. Milk contains 100 IU vitamin D per 250 ml; margarine contains 33 IU per tsp (5 ml). Remember, it is only milk that vitamin D is added to. Cheese, yogurt, ice cream and other dairy products are not fortified with vitamin D.

What about the safety of doses of vitamin D-3 in the range of 1000 IU – 4000 IU daily? The recommended intake for adults has been set much lower; 200 IU for adults over age 20; 400 IU for adults 51-70 years of age and 600 IU for adults over 70 years. Yet, much of the scientific literature points to a higher level of vitamin D for disease treatment and prevention. Vieth has written many articles and is emphatic that the "no observed adverse effect level (NOAEL) is at least 10,000 IU per day. He does state that levels of vitamin D of 40,000 IU per day would be a problem. Thus, a level of 4000 IU per day is perfectly safe. Vieth stresses that his recommendations are for vitamin D-3 (cholecalciferol) not vitamin D-2 or other forms of vitamin D.

It is six years now that I have taken vitamin D at 4000 IU or 100 micrograms or 0.1 milligrams per day, year round. My vitamin D still is only 99, which is considered optimal for helping minimize MS symptoms. I therefore suggest that you get with the program – sunshine plus supplementation.

Chapter 13

Emu Oil – A Natural Anti-inflammatory

Some of you will know that the funding for our first book was supported by emu oil sales. This is not the case with this book. Instead, I include emu oil for several different reasons.

Firstly, I believe that my daily intake (1 tsp or 5 ml) of emu oil was the first dietary supplement that helped my initial recovery. Oral emu oil seemed to enhance my energy – which was pitifully low for twelve or more months. As I thought about it, I came to believe emu oil's safe and natural anti-inflammatory effects were quite possibly the reasons for this enhanced well-being.

The Australian study by Snowden and Whitehouse (see References), showed that topical emu oil was more effective as an anti-inflammatory in wrist soreness and stiffness (arthritis) than a considerable dose of ibuprofen, a Non-Steroidal Anti Inflammatory Drug (NSAID). Lopez and his research team (see References) also demonstrated that emu oil was anti-inflammatory. In addition, there has never been any suggestion that emu oil slowed healing, as do NSAIDs. To the contrary, emu oil doubles the rate of wound healing and quadruples it relative to cortisone in a skin model of research, studied by Politis (see References).

It is now accepted that our body uses inflammation as part of the healing process, regardless of the organ, tissue or time of life. My understanding from this premise is that a similar type of healing occurs in our brain. In those of us with MS, neurons are injured by the white blood cells attacking their myelin sheath. During this process, free radicals are produced. The surrounding nerves, blood vessels and glial cells (astrocytes) sustain injury from these free radicals. While the glutathione, a potent antioxidant, quenches the free radicals, the emu oil may play a part in fine-tuning the healing response in the brain just as it does on the skin. This fine-tuning may speed the healing process and, in addition, reduce the local scarring as well.

Daily emu oil may provide this "injury reducing" anti-inflammatory effect whenever an MS flare-up occurs. I like to think of it as a very safe, natural, anti-inflammatory, perhaps reducing the need for cortisone steroid use when severe attacks occur. I now have a strong aversion to steroids, even though at one time I advocated their use as an anesthesiologist with considerable clinical practice experience. I believe that people with MS should avoid using oral or intravenous corticosteroids.

Despite thirty-five years of using corticosteroids (ACTH was an early form), doctors have never been able to prove or show that they have any lasting benefit to people with MS. To the contrary, physicians know that steroids can trigger occasional hip joint necrosis, can create early or premature cataracts and frequently can worsen osteoporosis. Hip joint necrosis is sometimes triggered by a single dose of corticosteroids. Somehow, the drug shuts down or blocks the blood supply to the joint lining. Once it dies, joint replacement is inevitable.

In all my years in medicine and now as an MS patient, physicians rarely say, "I have nothing to offer." If pushed, they will often fall back on corticosteroids, oral or intravenous. In all fairness, it is we patients who ask, "Can't you do something?!" If you have an acute MS flare-up, are blind and/or paralyzed and have no help or assistance to care for young children, you may have no recourse but to use corticosteroids. As a general rule, though, avoid them whenever possible.

Emu oil provides three other benefits. The first is skin care, a particular concern in a dry, low humidity climate such as Alberta or Colorado. For people with MS, reduced touch or skin sensation is common. This, plus dry, itchy skin, can be a poor combination. The moisturizing and healing effects of pure emu oil or a cream thereof, may delay, or even avoid skin tears, burns or pressure ulcers (bed sores).

Secondly, emu oil has the ability to relieve pain, both externally and internally. The pain relief of emu oil may be found with topical application or oral capsules or both. The most obvious example is shingles (herpes zoster, chicken pox or varicella in children). Topical application of emu oil can eliminate the pain from shingles for up to two hours. A reapplication works for another two hours and so on. As expected the blisters or scabs heal up faster. I believe this single therapy can reduce greatly, the likelihood of severe, ongoing "neuropathic" pain of post herpetic neuralgia. This pain syndrome afflicts at least five percent of shingles sufferers who respond poorly to oral medications. In fact, up to five percent of these people go on to commit suicide, the pain is so severe and all consuming. I believe this shingles neuropathic pain is similar to the neuropathic pain of MS. 70% of people with MS seek prescription medication for pain. Even a 20-50% reduction in this pain could improve our quality of life. Yes, I routinely take five, 500 mg emu oil capsules per day orally as a safe anti-inflammatory with some pain relief effect.

Similarly, when I have leg muscle spasms, I will apply a topical Joint Comfort mixture. This contains 20% emu oil plus glucosamine, MSM, boswellia, cetyl myristoleate (a fatty acid which assists soft tissue healing), devil's claw extract and peppermint. This mixture has helped many people with leg cramps and muscle spasms from MS. It works more often than I expect it to. The emu oil at 20% will have some direct benefits of its own and also act as a carrier through the skin the other compounds. (A recent study confirmed emu oil's ability to carry Vitamin E through the skin and raise the concentration of Vitamin E in the blood).

Finally, I thank the emu oil and the emu bird for important components of my personal health journey with MS. Our small acreage on Vancouver Island off the West Coast provided a healing milieu. Prominent in this was the emu life cycle, the beauty and peace of nature and my ability to look within for mind & spiritual issues. These combined with the increasing awareness of body, mind and spirit interaction, initiated some recovery from a progressive chronic illness.

In hindsight, I am grateful for being diagnosed with MS and leaving the hectic and near all-consuming life of academic medicine. My energy was consumed by teaching, research and clinical medicine. This left little time for key personal relationships with my family, and even my marriage. Sometimes I think I may not have recovered even a little if I had not looked outside regular neuroscience, "research only" based medicine. The west coast of North America, I feel, is one of the more enlightened cultures, climate, energy and geography on our planet earth. I am very grateful for this.

Chapter 14

Dietary Fat–
The Good and The Bad

Our brain is 60% fat. Hence the next time you are called a "fathead", take it as a compliment. Omega-3 fatty acids are by far the most important fats in brain development and function, healing and recovery. In this chapter, you will learn how and which fats should be in your foods and food supplements.

There are two essential fatty acids (EFAs) needed by humans. Omega-6 includes linoleic acid, gamma linolenic acid (GLA) and arachidonic acid (not from peanuts, which is arachidic acid). Omega-3, now thought to be the most essential fatty acid, is without doubt, the most important in our brain. The omega-3 family includes alpha-linolenic acid, DHA and EPA (see Figure 14.1). I will list sources, especially of omega-3, because almost everyone in North America is deficient in this one. Our intake of saturated fat must be moderate, and our trans fats near zero.

EFAs Made Simple:
EFAs play a role in every cell in the body. Their curved shape – like curves in a caterpillar—are absolutely critical for making healthy body cells including the brain cells called neurons and glia (astrocytes). If either Omega-6 or Omega-3 oils are hydrogenated, they become trans fatty

Fatty Acids Made Simple

The Omega-6 Family	The Omega-3 Family
Linoleic Acid (LA)	**Alpha-Linoleic Acid (ALA)**
(Found in Vegetable oils, seeds and nuts.)	(Found in green leafy vegetables, flax, flaxseed oil, hemp oil, canola oil, emu oil, walnuts, and Brazil nuts.)

Your body converts LA into: *Your body converts ALA into:*

↓ ↓

Gamma-Linolenic Acid (GLA)	**Eicosapentaenoic Acid (EPA)**
(GLA is also found in borage and primrose oil.)	(EPA is also found in fish oil)

Your body converts GLA into: *Your body converts EPA into:*

↓ ↓

Arachidonic Acid (AA)	**Docosahexaenoic Acid (DHA)**
(AA is also found in meat.)	(DHA is also found in fish oil.)

↓ ↓

| **The Omega-6 Family of Eicosanoids**
 Unhappy or Inflammatory
 Prostaglandins | **The Omega-3 Family of Eicosanoids**
 Happy or Anti-inflammatory
 Prostaglandins |

Figure 14.1 *Adapted from: The Omega Diet by a Simopoulos, M.D. & J. Robinson Harper Perennial, 1999, p. 40.*

acids.[1] Trans fats tend to be straight and they greatly reduce the normal health and function of every cell, including brain cells. We have had trans fats from hydrogenated oils in our diet for over 50 years. Shortening, hard margarine, baked goods and deep-frying oils (i.e. for frying potato chips) usually contain trans fats. You must learn to read labels, for your own protection and long-term health. Remember, all our body's cells are gradually changed and replaced over time. Hence, healing is possible even in the brain and spinal cord.

I routinely read food labels, even those on my chocolate bars in order to avoid all "modified", "hydrogenated" or "trans" fats. All of these names denote trans fats. Identification gets easier all the time, as awareness increases. In fact, manufacturers are now using "No Trans Fats" as a marketing tool. This is a great help. Similarly, I do not order restaurant or take-out food which has been deep-fried or which has had trans fats used in its baking process. Pay attention to the choice of your salad dressings. If you are in doubt use olive oil, high in monounsaturated fats, and a vinaigrette choice. Saturated fats, in moderation only, are **much safer** than trans fats. In fact, our bodies can make MUFAs out of certain saturated fats. For cooking, Denise and I use butter, but if high heat is needed, i.e. deep-frying, we suggest coconut, peanut or palm oil. When I was in France in late 2003 at the International Fats and Oil Congress, I learned that they are well ahead of North Americans. One of the major oil suppliers to France claimed all of their chips (French fries) were cooked without trans fat oils! I was impressed.

My hope is that you now understand that trans fats are the very bad fats. Saturated fats and liquid oils, if they are used in moderation are the very good fats. Liquid oils contain

---

1. Hydrogenation is a process which converts a liquid oil to a solid fat. In this process, heat and hydrogen gas are added to the liquid oil. The chemical reaction, which occurs, adds hydrogen atoms to the oil and the oil becomes solid.

monounsaturated (MUFA)[2] and polyunsaturated (PUFA) fat, which are generally considered as healthy fats. However, I want to specify which PUFAs are most important to people with MS, or to those who have other inflammations in their body. This includes ALS (Amyotrophic Lateral Sclerosis or Lou Gehrig's Disease), fibromyalgia, arthritis (osteo, rheumatoid), psoriasis, asthma, Meniere's, Parkinson's, lupus, chronic fatigue syndrome and all other inflammatory conditions. In fact, it is now thought that inflammation occurs in every disease process. Please refer to the Omega-6 and Omega-3 pathways diagram (Figure 14.1). You will note each pathway has a Family of Eicosanoids (or prostaglandins) at the bottom. These are designed to counterbalance one another.

Please remember almost all of the unhappy or unpleasant prostaglandins are at the end of the Omega-6 pathway. These are the ones that trigger the inflammation associated with arthritis, asthma, menstrual cramps, hay fever (allergic rhinitis), the swelling of the nerves in MS or the joint inflammation in arthritis attacks, and the inflammation associated with degenerative diseases.

Unfortunately, at least 80% of us in North America have much more Omega-6 in our diet than Omega-3. We consume nearly 20 times more omega-6 fats than omega-3 fats. Consequently, we suffer from an excess of the Omega-6 "unhappy" eicosanoids or prostaglandins. Why is this so? We are victims of our own shopping preferences. We have a huge selection of processed and packaged foods in our grocery stores—crackers, cookies, cake mixes, sauces, dips and baked goods and more. These usually contain vegetable oils that are high in Omega-6 fat. Furthermore, these veg-

---

2. Fat contains long chains of carbon atoms. Attached to the carbon atoms are oxygen and hydrogen. When a fat holds all the hydrogen that it can, it is called a saturated fat. Butter, lard and coconut oil are all saturated. They are also solid fats. If a fat has room for one more hydrogen, it is monounsaturated. Olive oil, canola oil and peanut oil are monounsaturated fats (MUFAs) and are liquid. If a fat has room for 2 or more hydrogen atoms, it is a polyunsaturated fat. Corn oil and safflower oils are polyunsaturated fats (PUFAs) and liquid.

etable oils have been modified or hydrogenated, resulting in harmful trans fats.

We expect any product to be odorless, or at least, not to smell rancid. Hence, the rampant marketing and sales of not only trans fats, but also of oils high in Omega-6 fatty acids. Omega-6 oils keep much better on the store shelf than do the Omega-3 oils. Have you ever seen a flax margarine, flax cooking oil or even flax salad oil? No. This is why: flax oil is high in Omegra-3 fatty acids and has a short shelf life. Similarly, fish oils are very high in Omega-3 fatty acids. Omega-3 fatty acids easily breakdown and become rancid. This explains the relative unpopularity of taking a spoonful of cod liver oil and many fish oils – they can have a strong odor and flavor.

What about the long-touted evening primrose oil, or more recent, borage oil, for multiple sclerosis? Despite three decades of studies testing these in MS, we have no confirming studies of note. I will suggest why this conundrum has occurred.

Evening primrose oil and borage oil contain GLA, which belongs to the Omega-6 family. Converting linoleic acid (Omega-6) to GLA and alpha-linolenic acid (Omega-3) to EPA requires the same enzyme. (See Figure 14.1). By adding more GLA, less of the enzyme is needed for converting linoleic acid to GLA. This leaves more of the enzyme available for converting alpha-linolenic acid to EPA and DHA, two key brain fats. However, most people's diets are very low in alpha-linolenic acid. Therefore, only a small amount of alpha-linoleic can be converted to EPA and the benefits would be minimal.

GLA supplementation is generally not advised. According to Franco Cavaleri, GLA supplementation can "fuel more disease if unhealthy dietary habits aren't changed at the same time." (p. 258). GLA can be converted to arachidonic acid in the cells. Arachidonic acid can then be transformed into prostaglandins that promote inflammation. As mentioned previously, many of our diseases also have inflammation associated with them. Therefore, we would not want to add to the inflammation process by increasing GLA. It is recommended that anyone supplementing with borage oil or evening primrose oil should also take a fish oil supplement. This will reduce arachidonic acid production and subsequent inflammation.

A wealth of studies support the health benefits of omega-3 fats. They play an important role in brain health, heart health, skin health, immune function, joint mobility and protection against inflammation and cancer. The omega-3 parent, alpha-linolenic acid, is found in plant sources. The richest sources are flax, hemp, canola, soybean and walnut. The alpha-linolenic acid can then be converted to EPA and DHA. Fish oil is a rich source of EPA and DHA.

Unfortunately, the conversion of alpha-linolenic acid to DHA is limited. Much of the dietary alpha-linolenic acid is oxidized and, on average, only 3.8% becomes EPA which is then converted to DHA. In addition, a deficiency in zinc, magnesium, vitamin C, vitamin B-3 or vitamin B-6 will impair conversion to EPA and production of the "happy" prostaglandins. Because our diets contain so little alpha-linoleic acid, and limited EPA is produced from it, a more efficient way to get EPA and DHA is from fish oil supplements. Indeed, research has shown that EPA increases more in body cells when a fish oil supplement is given with dietary alpha-linolenic acid.

The use of fish oils and the fact that they contain high amounts of EPA and DHA merits special mention. EPA and DHA are particularly important in the first year of human life for our ongoing brain development. EPA and DHA are essential at this time, and breast milk is still considered the best source. The mother can enhance the amount of Omega-3s in her breast milk by taking a good Omega-3 supplement. Similarly, infant formulas should have the Omega-3 oils added to them. In most countries this has already occurred. DHA has just recently been added to infant formula in Canada.

More recently, krill oil has been combined with fish oils. Krill oil comes from a tiny shrimp-like creature which is an important food source for whales, penguins and fish. Krill oil is rich in EPA and DHA and has powerful antioxidants such as vitamin A, vitamin E and astaxathin. The antioxidant activity in krill oil is 550 times more potent than vitamin E alone. The ratio of Omega-3:Omega-6 is extremely high, 30:1. Furthermore, krill oil has a high level of phospholipids, which are vital to brain function, spinal cord and nerves. Most fish oils do not provide these phospholipids. Krill oil not only provides unique brain health benefits, but also a more concentrated amount of EPA and DHA.

Two potential downsides of fish and fish oils are their cost and the toxins they carry. In recent recommendations, most of us should eat canned tuna only once a week – due to the heavy metals, dioxins and other contaminants in the tuna. Similarly, farmed salmon can contain significant levels of toxins depending on the location it is farmed and the type of feed and origin of the feed. For example, salmon originating from the North Sea (above Europe) has a reasonably high toxic load and this salmon is best eaten only once a month. Salmon farmed in North America can best be eaten every two weeks. Finally, salmon farmed off Chile in South America can safely be eaten once a week. These are only recommendations and will vary according to your use of safe, healthy detoxification choices—namely taking glutathione-building blocks of bioactive cysteine and/or infrared sauna with sand emitter in the 6-20 micron range. Detoxification by ingesting bioactive cysteine and by infrared sauna is discussed in Chapters 11 and 8, respectively.

Toxicity and taste issues of fish oils can be overcome by purchasing fish oils which have undergone a purification process. Ensure that you buy quality, pharmaceutical grade fish oils. Increased cost is the downside of this. Always keep in mind that cold-water fish is higher in the healthy Omega-3 fats than warm water fish. Similarly, krill oil has a high level of Omega-3s and is perhaps superior to fish oil because it has a higher level of DHA and also contains beneficial phospholipids for brain health. The downside of krill oil is that it is expensive.

I strongly recommend flax as a source of omega-3s for a host of reasons. Firstly, it is safe, as it has no fish-related heavy metals and dioxins, and secondly, it is the least expensive source of Omega-3 fat. One to two tablespoons of ground flax seed provides 1.8 – 3.6 g alpha-linolenic acid. This meets the adequate intake of alpha-linolenic acid for adults.

Thirdly, ground flax is 25% soluble and 75% insoluble fiber. This high fiber content has a great "brush, brush" cleansing ability within our large bowel. In addition, the fiber absorbs toxins from the bowel, including those excreted in the bile. For example, drug reabsorption is lowered, as are heavy metals and the "bad" cholesterol, LDL or Low Density Lipoprotein. Fourthly, flax's rich brown seed-coat contains lignans which reduce our risk of bowel cancer, breast cancer, prostate cancer and the risk of heart attack and stroke as well. Considering the three causes of death in North America are heart disease, cancer and stroke respectively, we should take advantage of all these benefits of flax. The fiber is also a useful asset to many of us with MS as we tend toward constipation.

An important side note here is that flax is acceptable to people with celiac disease. For those who are truly allergic to flax, the next best option is ground hemp or hemp oil. Allergic reactions to both hemp and flax are fortunately quite uncommon. Hemp is a two to one ratio of Omega-6 to Omega-3 and also has a reasonable amount of GLA (gamma linolenic acid, an Omega-6 fat). This is good news for those of you who are already using GLA and who would rather "fight than switch". (Remember to also take a fish oil supplement.)

An easy option is to eat 2-3 tablespoons of ground flax (30-45 ml) every day. It can be added to hot cereal (oatmeal), cold cereal, salads, muffins, breads (made with grains which you can tolerate), or even spread on toast. Whole flax seed keeps well for many months. Once flax is ground in a coffee grinder or kitchen blender, it keeps well for several weeks. I usually grind enough for a week to ten days and then store it in a cool place. Refrigeration is fine, but not necessary. Make sure you add flax to your diet daily, as a habit.

Even though people often say "you must use it in the next 20-30 minutes after grinding", I suggest that this is a bit "over the top". It will not lose its freshness that quickly. For those who cannot or choose not to have ground flax, flax oil is an option. However it will not have the fiber and lignan advantages of ground flax. Flax oil comes in bottles or capsules and must be stored in the refrigerator to prevent it from going rancid.

For any post-menopausal women who have hot flashes or "power surges", flax has significant phytoestrogens. These are the equivalent of soy phytoestrogens and are an excellent alternative for those concerned about excess soy in their diet.

Another important issue to address is the "cyano" or cyanide factor with flax. This is no problem whatsoever and is well addressed in the superb book on flax, "Flaxseed in Human Nutrition". On page 26, the expert, J.K. Daun informs us that when the cyanide equivalent is calculated in, an adult can consume more than one kilogram (2.2 lb) per day before exhibiting acute cyanic toxicity.

In summary, ground flax intake of 30-45 mls (2-3 tablespoons) per day is very high on my "Top Ten Choices" list. Flax grown in cool areas such as northern Europe, South Australia or Western Canada is the highest in polyunsaturated fatty acids. Ensure adequate amounts of EPA and DHA by taking fish oil supplements. Although eating fish several times a week will provide the required omega-3s, this is not recommended because of toxins. Rely on a combination of flax and purified fish oils to meet your Omega-3 needs.

The optimal amount of Omega-3 for health is still being investigated. Health Canada recommends 1.6g/day alpha-linolenic acid for adult men and 1.1g/day for adult women. Studies have shown that 900 mg/day of fish oil has a positive impact on mortality rates in patients with heart disease. This amount of fish oil can be obtained from eating salmon 5 times per week, or herring 3 times per week. A standard fish oil supplement provides 300 mg Omega-3 fat per capsule.

Dr. Bruce Holub from the University of Guelph, Ontario, is one of Canada's leading experts on essential fatty acids. Through his research, he recommends the following amounts of Omega-3 fatty acids: 300 mg / day for pregnant and breastfeeding women, 650 mg / day for healthy adults and, 900-1000 mg / day for people with heart disease.

The evidence for eliminating trans fats, reducing Omega-6 fats and increasing Omega-3 fats is overwhelming. Evaluate the fats in your diet. Then, make the necessary changes so that your diet includes the healthy fats every day. It will be a positive step in your health journey!

Chapter 15

These Are A Few Of My Favourite Things

I have structured this chapter to include helpful hints or tips for enhancing your coping skills and increasing your happiness while controlling your multiple sclerosis or other chronic illness. I will start with the top of the body (brain) and work on down to a potpourri of "short snappers" of unrelated tips.

Natural Stress Management:
To begin, let us consider brain issues. Depression has been dealt with in Chapter 6 on depression. First, let me mention a completely natural dietary supplement, which helps the body resist stress. It is a tiny protein having a 10 amino acid ring. (See **www.emu.ca.**)

This product was first patented in France and is now available in many countries worldwide. Countries in which it is available include Canada, U.S.A., Australia and many Asian countries. This 10 amino acid ring is derived from milk and acts on the GABA receptor in the brain. This is the same receptor that works with valerian or the benzodiazepine drugs such as Valium, Seran, Ativan, and Librium. This peptide, like the drugs mentioned, relieves anxiety. Happily this milk compound is non-addicting, does not suppress dream sleep (REM) and does not worsen our pain tolerance. All of the benzodiazepines have these disadvantages and, hence, are best avoided in MS and most other brain injuries or illnesses. One to three capsules of this food, or nutraceutical, can reduce anxiety and can help improve sleep.

Melatonin, is another dietary supplement readily available in the USA and some other countries. Our body makes melatonin adequately on its own as long as two guidelines are followed. Firstly, we have better quality sleep and produce more melatonin if we are in a totally dark room. Secondly, we need at least 15-20 minutes of bright, full-spectrum light per day to stimulate melatonin production in our body. One option is to purchase a "Seasonal Affective Disorder" (SAD) light and spend 15-20 minutes in front of it daily. Exposure to sunlight on a bright or sunny day will do this equally well. However, some of us live in quite cloudy areas, are unable to get outside during the day, or sit near a sunny window. In fact, studies have documented that people who work by a window, have 7% improved productivity. An inexpensive alternative to a SAD light is to get a full spectrum light (usually fluorescent light, as needed to grow plants) and sit under this for 2-3 hours a day. I have seen this help a number of folks on the West Coast of Canada (see **www.emu.ca** for resources). As usual, I prefer to let our body produce melatonin with as little drug or supplement as possible. However, you decide what is best for you. It is your journey, not mine or anyone else's!

A Natural Solution for Energy, Brain Fog and Migraines:
My favorite energy drink is an herbal tonic that contains ginseng, gingko biloba, chamomile, damiana, angelica and other herbs. (See **www.emu.ca**.) In addition, this herbal tonic contains guarana—the most popular soft drink additive in Brazil. Research on guarana reveals its long use by the native people of the Amazon rain forest. Evidence suggests its use for relieving fatigue, boosting energy, aiding concentration and brightening mood.

Guarana contains guaranine, a chemical substance with effects similar to caffeine. Yet, a dose of this tonic is equal to only 100 mgs of caffeine, which is less than one cup of regular coffee. Even better, guarana gives 6-8 hours of slow burn, without the classic roller-coaster effects that many of us experience with coffee, tea or cola drinks. I feel jangled after drinking something with caffeine. You could consider this to reduce your caffeine intake or as a "brain fog" remedy.

I usually take one ounce (30 ml) of this tonic every day. It immediately helps to boost potassium and magnesium in the body, and these increase alertness. Some people use this tonic twice a day. However, many of us will prefer to limit ourselves to one drink a day, to minimize caffeine side effects, like diarrhea, or stomach upset. I use this early in the day, or before 3:00 p.m., so that I can sleep fine at night. I usually take a half dose (15 ml) before I exercise – it improves my stamina and I get a better workout. Although the tonic is best taken early in the day, I will take another dose at a later time, even at night, to "break" or stop a migraine.

For the longest time I avoided taking this tonic later in the day, as I tolerate caffeine poorly and have trouble sleeping. One evening I had a nasty migraine headache and took only my ordinary, over-the-counter medications such as dimenhydrate, (Gravol), acetominophen (paracetamol) and ibuprofen. Denise had seen me improve previous headaches by using this tonic, which boosts potassium and magnesium quickly. When she asked, now at 10:30 at night, "Why don't you try the tonic?" I replied, "I want to be able to get to sleep tonight." She sagely stated, "Well, you're not able to sleep now, are you?" I relented, and in fifteen minutes, my headache was much better and I was asleep twenty minutes later!

Migraine troubles are worth discussing in a book about MS, because 80% of people with MS also suffer from these headaches. My first line of defense against migraines is to avoid the foods to which I am sensitive. My number one nemesis is wheat, wheat flour and wheat pasta. As I previously wrote, I discovered my wheat intolerance as a result of drinking wheat-based beer. I realize this is not totally scientific, but as I learned more about lectins and the "Stone Age Diet", this made considerable sense.

Constipation Solutions:

Prevention is number one. There is no such thing as "too much fiber". Ground flax, is my all-time favourite, but psyllium, whole grains and beans help too! Magnesium salts can be an effective option. If cost is a huge issue, take 1/2 teaspoon or 2.5 mls of magnesium sulfate (Epsom salts) in a glass of water, by mouth, and stay near a washroom or toilet. Plenty of good water, daily, is still very useful. Insist on eight glasses a day (250 mls each or 8oz) and aim for twelve!

Warm Mineral Baths for Muscle Relaxation:

Try a warm bath before bed, with bath salts, including a handful of magnesium sulfate (Epsom salts). This will have several benefits. It will relax you and your muscles and perhaps even the sensors in your peripheral nerves. Hopefully, this will minimize the dreaded pains and muscle spasms so common in people with MS, especially during the night. I "discovered" the value of Epsom salt baths from my European-trained massage therapist, Isabella, prior to a two-day-bicycle event for MS called the "Grape Escape" (see **www.emu.ca** for links to this MS Canada event, on Vancouver Island, B.C.) Riding in this event also increased my enthusiasm for my energy tonic as after four hours of cycling it reduced my groin muscle spasm and enabled me to lift my leg easily over my bicycle seat to mount and dismount!

Digestive Enzymes:

Please do not interpret this as a solution just for "old people". By the age of 40, most of us start to reduce our stomach acid secretion. This reduced acid decreases the pre-digestion of our food. In addition, production of our regular enzymes (gall bladder, bile and pancreas) declines with age. The end result is that our ability to recover nutrients from food is impaired. Hence, reasonable use of digestive enzymes will allow us to digest and absorb nutrients more effectively from whole foods and minimize other gastrointestinal symptoms. A good digestive enzyme will include lactase (acts on sugar in milk), lipase (acts on fat), and protease (acts on protein).

Some enzymes also contain betaine hydrochloride to increase stomach acid. Enhanced digestion can decrease or eliminate heartburn, gas (burps or farts, too!), diarrhea, constipation and should maximize nutrient absorption from our diet. I much prefer the plant digestive enzymes to drugs for heartburn, as drugs reduce or even eliminate acid secretion. This then markedly reduces our normal digestive ability. See **www.emu.ca** for two or more choices of digestive enzymes.

Chocolate – Especially Dark Chocolate:

I admit I am a "recovering chocoholic"! The lipase in the digestive enzymes permits me to enjoy one or two or, occasionally, three, chocolates. Chocolate is a "mood elevator". For me, it is a sign that I need to "top up" my emotional energy and/or, "slow down". Dark chocolate is "the best", hands down! It is full of beneficial antioxidants. But, remember, read the labels to avoid those harmful trans (hydrogenated or modified) fats. Butter, palm oil or coconut oil, in moderation, are better for health. Beware of the calories in chocolate — fat provides 9 calories per gram, as opposed to 4 calories per gram for protein and for carbohydrates. Also, watch out for liqueur chocolates – alcohol provides 7 calories per gram, and many of these chocolates are especially sweet. Use chocolate as an occasional treat. Weight gain tends to be a problem with people as they age. This can be even more of a problem for people who are not very active or with physical limitations because of MS.

Probiotics and Prebiotics:

Our gut contains about 1-2 kilograms of friendly bacteria. These beneficial bacteria, such as Lactobacillus acidophilus and Bifidobacterium bifidum are known as probiotics. These bacteria produce substances that promote the health of the cells lining the bowel. Too, these bacteria influence our general health. They inhibit the growth of harmful bacteria, increase our resistance to infection and aid the immune system.

Traditionally, yoghurt and fermented foods have been used for hundreds, if not thousands of years, to supply our bodies with probiotic bacteria. People eating a poor diet or suffering from diarrhea can be deficient in probiotic bacteria. Some drugs, especially antibiotics and some hormones, upset this natural process. A minimum use of probiotics would be advisable with hormone therapy such as estrogen (e.g. oral contraceptive or hormone replacement therapy) and drugs such as cortisone. People are advised to take probiotics following antibiotics in order to re-populate the gut with friendly bacteria.

A daily source of probiotics from food or supplements is recommended. This can be especially important while traveling and being exposed to different bacteria in food or the environment. In addition, minimize eating any food that causes diarrhea or loose stools. This is important because the beneficial bacteria can be flushed out of the body. For me, these foods to avoid include fat, milk, lactose, legumes, beans and beer because they all promote gastric hurry. Scientists claim that the food or probiotic supplement should supply from 1 million to 1 billion live bacteria in order to be effective. See **www.emu.ca** for probiotic choices.

Prebiotics are "food" for the friendly bacteria, to optimize their healthy synergy with us. These include fructo-oligocaccarides such as inulin, which cannot be digested or absorbed by humans. I believe these are most useful if one is having trouble recovering from almost any bowel upset. This would include irritable bowel syndrome (IBS), a viral or gastro-intestinal infection, dysentery, diverticulitis, bowel polyps or preparation for surgery or radiology.

Calcium and Magnesium:

Calcium, zinc, manganese and Vitamin K are all important to slow down or even reverse osteoporosis. Build your calcium intake, therefore, on a good multi-vitamin / multi-mineral base. Take at least half as much magnesium per day as calcium. Denise and I believe the easiest calcium to absorb is that derived from milk, in the form of calcium phosphate (see **www.emu.ca**). Next best sources of calcium are calcium citrate and calcium lactate. I currently aim for 2,000 mgs of elemental calcium per day. Absorption is best when timed with food, in 500 mgs per meal or snack, as acidity improves absorption.

I focus on this much calcium because I have early osteoporosis in my spine and the earliest stage of osteopenia in my legs. This has progressed (worsened) over the last six years since my leg fracture in 1998, when my legs and spine were both osteopenic. This is in spite of my boost in vitamin D for six years of 4,000 IU per day; hence, my emphasis on calcium and magnesium. Any of us, especially those of us with MS, who are not mobile or physically active, are sitting ducks for osteoporosis. I suggest you get evaluated for bone density and be proactive against osteoporosis.

My primary source of calcium phosphate is only one-tenth magnesium so I often take a magnesium supplement with the calcium, too. In addition, my modest physical recovery adds to the amount of walking and weight bearing I can do. Hence, mobility is a further benefit because it will slow down your osteoporosis as well. Please remember, any corticosteroid use speeds up osteoporosis in anyone who uses it. So, think about the effects on your bones before you decide to take corticosteroids.

Infrared Sauna:
I outlined this in my chapter on detoxification. I mention it again not only to affirm my confidence in it but also to urge you to start slowly. My infrared sauna teacher advised me to start at the lower temperatures and only 10-15 minutes every second day. Well, of course, I "knew better", and went for 30-35 minutes per day at upper temperatures on alternating days for a week. This caused very low energy days and was accompanied by a poor quality brain-thinking. I went too far, too fast. I took a week off from the sauna and am working forward much more slowly. The benefits of reducing toxins, probably enhanced cardiac fitness and even weight loss while sitting on my butt, will be worth the slow start-up!

Music:

Enjoyment of music has been life long for me. However, now I also think of it for its therapeutic effects of relaxation, stress reduction, training back-up brain pathways and even improving my breathing control and speech for the long term. My newest passion is learning to play the Irish harp and eventually sing along with it. I have chosen the harp as it will enhance my finger dexterity and also optimize forming new motor pathways. Some of my favourite songs are Celtic or country ballads. I believe any musical instrument is helpful, but especially the voice. To sing, we do best if we are rested, focused and feeling well emotionally. Each of these is an important reminder for maintaining a balance in my life.

Future endeavours I recommend: 1) Horse back riding. This can be Western, English or Therapeutic style. I love Winston Churchill's quote, "Time spent with a horse is never wasted." 2) Time spent with a dog. I believe this is both man and woman's best friend, as our dog will always forgive us; and 3) Dance. Watch the movie, "Shall We Dance" as motivation to dance. Then, get to know yourself and your partner better!

This then is an overview of some of the things I feel are important to help one cope with chronic illness. Also, some of these items can add a great deal of joy to life. Perhaps you, too, have tips or ideas that promote health and improve the quality of your life. If so, enjoy!

Chapter 16

Our 5 Senses and Position Sense (Proprioception)

Hearing is, of course, supplied by a "double" nerve – balance and auditory. The "balance component" or, "semicircular canals" affects many of us with MS. I can now look back on a day with my kids at an amusement park outside Calgary. I rode the Himalayan with my sons, Warren and Brian. The ride went round and round, and up and down. I not only got nauseated and had wobbly knees, but this condition persisted for twelve hours. In retrospect, I believe this persistence and easy nausea, which increased in my thirties, was likely MS. When I met a woman with MS from Washington State, USA, intractable nausea was her most challenging symptom. I can empathize with her. Many of us with MS believe that our problem with balance is also associated with this nerve. Instead, it may also be related to our loss of proprioception, that is, knowing where our limbs are in relation to our body. We become very eye or vision dependent when we begin to lose our balance.

Hearing is not as frequently affected in MS as vestibular or semicircular canal balance. However, it is not uncommon during an MS attack, to be hypersensitive to hearing, so that any sound jangles us. Jangles, I realize, is not a medical term. What I mean is that certain sounds or even rhythms seem to acutely irritate us and can make us very uncomfortable with our surroundings. This, too, is a hypersensitivity, where the hearing mechanism is not blunted but is more irritable than normal. My newest toy to reduce unpleasant noise is a special pair of headphones with Acoustic Noise Cancelling properties. They are superb on airplanes and even in your dentist's chair. They cancel out much of the unpleasant sound and yet they still permit conversation. These have been a great asset if travelling in noisy surroundings, as they secondarily reduce fatigue resulting from the noise.

Denise and I have a good friend, Gill, who has major hearing problems with MS. She is a nurse and is nearly deaf, due to MS injury to both inner ears (the acoustic collecting nerve within the brain). In fact, this must be exceedingly rare, for upon review by an experienced MS neurologist, she was referred, expeditiously, to an Ear, Nose & Throat (ENT) specialist. This ENT specialist examined her, repeated her MRI and reassured her it was definitely due to her MS. The most striking feature of this is that the MS neurologist had given Gill the same referral, with the same ENT surgeon, with the same outcome, two to three years earlier!

Hearing is also one of our earliest sensations. Good quality hearing is developed much before vision becomes dominant. This might explain our acoustic expertise in water, a skill we share with our fellow mammals, such as dolphins and whales. For decades, operating room personnel have been taught that hearing is often our last sense to disappear and our first to come back under anesthesia. Making positive comments about the person "asleep", makes for better healing, less pain and quicker recovery than making negative ones. Unfortunately, negative comments and jokes about obesity are, in my anesthesiology experience, common.

I have great empathy for Gill and others who have hearing loss. My Dad, who sustained a measure of hearing loss in World War II, would often debate with me the importance of hearing versus vision. Over several years I accepted that the greater loss would be hearing loss.

Hearing problems can be assisted by a number of physical devices. Also, the health of our nerve cells in the inner ear can be helped by improvement in our antioxidants, especially glutathione. Music is an underused option for recovery that we can try. We know that different types of music are pleasant or unpleasant to us individually. In addition, music by Mozart, has been shown to calm the brain (even to an alpha rhythm), like meditation, to enhance learning. When my hearing is hypersensitive or "jangled", it is usually "classical" music that works best for me. This can even include the different tonic sounds of Asia or India. If I focus on learning music, via playing tuba, tenor saxophone or voice, I believe I am helping my brain recruit new pathways. My newest goal in music now is to play the Irish harp, and to sing with it too!

Voice is probably the most challenging of all our senses, as our personal breathing, vocal cord position, emotion, and mouth muscles are all involved in speech. When my brother Stewart, a singer and musician, died in 1994, my grief at his loss made it nearly impossible for me to sing for almost a year. I believe music can be a very useful tool to help enhance our mind, body and spirit connection. In addition, optimal breathing can help not just our singing voice, but also can significantly help improve our speech in MS in the long-term. Working with music's pitch and tone stimulates hearing. This, in turn, will help our speech. Choir lessons will much improve our breathing patterns to protect our speaking abilities. Yoga is quite helpful as well.

Taste is another of our five senses. In fact, we have only four major taste buds (sweet, sour, bitter and salty) and five minor ones. This relative lack of taste buds further reminds me of the importance of planning a well-balanced diet with supplements. We can not rely solely on taste to ensure that we meet our nutrient needs. We are programmed, by evolution, to enjoy fat and sweet. However, a diet of doughnuts and french fries does not provide us with all the nutrients for health. Sometimes, too, we crave foods. Pica is the extreme in craving – people with pica have been known to eat clay or to chew relentlessly on ice cubes. It is thought that pica might be the body's response to a nutrient deficiency. For example, the ice craving usually declines with iron supplementation.

In contrast to our limited taste buds, dogs and horses have some 200 taste buds and cows and emus are felt to have 500! Hence, unlike animals, humans cannot instinctively search out needed nutrients important to survival. We need to plan to eat a variety of foods every day. Thus, wisdom and nutrition education can be very helpful to people so that they have the right balance of foods and supplements to optimize our health and recovery from MS or other chronic diseases.

Taste is essential for our enjoyment of food. Anything interfering with our sense of smell can result in a diminished sense of taste. Thus, taste and smell are closely linked. In addition, many drugs can interfere with our ability to taste and smell foods. Some drugs can alter how foods taste. Other drugs may decrease saliva and cause a loss of taste sensation. So, be aware of any changes in taste or smell when you take new medications and report them to your doctor. People who have changes in taste or smell often eat less. A reduced food intake might cause inadequate intake of important nutrients.

Even though the sense of smell is perhaps our oldest and longest established sense, it is the one we rarely consider in regular Western medicines. It should be recognized that there is a wide spectrum of smelling abilities – there are super-sniffers, average sniffers and minimal sniffers. When I smell certain irritating or pungent, unpleasant smells, I often make tracks to avoid them. Whenever I ignore this sensation, I often pay dearly for it with a migraine headache. And, I do not believe that recurrent migraines are a particularly good thing for the long-term well-being of our brain.

One smell I cannot tolerate is that of a "self-cleaning oven" heating at its characteristic, high temperature. Not only do I avoid and grump about the smell, but Denise will try and do this when I am away from home.

The upside of our sense of smell is that there are also pleasant smells. Aromatherapy is commonly practiced in Europe and on the west coast of North America, and is spreading to all parts of the globe. I now accept that this is more than just an incredible perfume or "Scent of a Woman", but, in fact, it has some safe, simple advantages for those of us with MS.

Aromatherapy, is an ancient form of healing using pure essential oils extracted from flowers, leaves, petals, blossoms, bark, trees, roots, twigs, seeds, berries, resins and rinds. The oils are very powerful, effective, and are what gives the plants their fragrance. These highly volatile oils are sensitive to heat and light, contain hormones and vitamins, are soluble in alcohol and oil, and are not water-soluble.

Acting on the central nervous system, essential oils stimulate the body's natural ability to heal itself, balance the body, and to rejuvenate & calm mind, body and spirit. These essential oils can be administered through massage, in baths or showers, and as room fragrances.

Some randomized controlled trials have suggested that the oils of certain flowers (like lavender) may have antidepressant and anti-anxiety properties. Aromatherapy is an effective complementary therapy for helping to manage chronic pain.

"Essential oils are like a team of good friends, all helping out in the best way they can when their particular attributes are needed."[3]

"In ancient Greece aromatic oils were often employed for their sleep inducing, antidepressant or aphrodisiac properties, and it was recognized that certain odours could improve mental alertness and aid concentration."[4]

Before leaving aromatherapy I would like to include one more plant, namely cistus ladaniferus. French aromatherapy experts particularly recommend this essential oil for reducing the fatigue of MS. I am working on trying this out personally. Watch our website, **www.emu.ca**, for further updates.

---

3. The Fragrant Pharmacy, Valerie Ann Worwood, p. 98, Bantam Books, 1993.
4. Aromatherapy for Everyone, Tisserand, Robert, 1988.

METHODS OF APPLICATION

METHOD OF APPLICATION	DROPS OF ESSENTIAL OIL	AMOUNT OF CARRIER OIL OR WATER
Massage (full body)	10 to 15 drops	25 ml / 1 oz oil
Massage (localized area)	15-20 drops	10 ml carrier oil
Bath	6-10 drops	1 tsp carrier oil in full tub of water
Inhalation (steam)	3-5 drops	Bowl of boiled water
Inhalation (tissue)	2-3 drops	n/a
Diffuser	6-8 drops	Water as required
Room Sprayer	10-15 drops	100 ml water
Compress	4-6 drops	Bowl of water

If you are interested in learning more about aromatherapy, essential oil applications and which oils to use, I suggest you do your research and/or consult an aromatherapist before beginning your adventure with essential oils.

NOTE: It is important to purchase 100% pure essential oils from a reputable supplier.

On Friday, 10 September 2004, at the British Psychological Society's Division of Health Psychology Annual Conference in Edinburgh, new research by psychologists revealed the positive effects of aromatherapy on the quality of life for Multiple Sclerosis (MS) sufferers. These researchers, at the University of Teeside, in Middlesbrough, England, found MS patients, in spite of experiencing the same symptoms, felt more vitality, happiness and peace during aromatherapy treatment, and less depression, fatigue and anxiety. The authors say that the mechanism by which improvements in quality of life occurred is unknown, but that there is «growing evidence for the effectiveness of aromatherapy on chronic illness». This finding offers some hope that whilst a cure is sought for chronic illness, Health Psychology could help people to live with its effects in the long-term.[5]

---

5. The British Psychological Society (BPS), Essential Hope for Multiple Sclerosis, Division of Health Psychology, BPS Press Office, 17 September 2004; Ref. PR645

PSYCHO-AROMATHERAPY

ESSENTIAL	APHRODISIAC		REGULATING		EUPHORIC		MEMORY/MENTAL STIMULANT		SEDATIVE		INVIGORATING	
OILS	Clary Sage	Jasmine	Bergamot	Frankincense	Clary Sage	Grapefruit	Black Pepper	Lemon	Chamomile	Lavender	Cardamom	Clary Sage
	Patchouli	Ylang Ylang	Geranium	Rosewood	Jasmine	Rose Otto	Peppermint	Rosemary	Marjoram	Orange	Lemongrass	Patchouli
Type of Problems Relieved	Emotional Coldness, Shyness, Impotence, Frigidity.		Anxiety with Depression, Mood Swings, Menstrual or Menopausal Imbalance.		Depression, Moodiness, Lack of Confidence.		Mental Fatigue, Difficulty in Concentrating, Poor Memory.		Anxiety, Stress, Hypertension, Insomnia, Anger, Irritability.		Boredom, Lethargy, Immune Deficiency.	
Neurochemical Secreted	ENDORPHINS		VARIOUS		ENKEPHALINS		VARIOUS		SEROTONIN		NORADRENALINE	
Part of Brain Triggered By Essential Oil	PITUITARY		HYPOTHALAMUS		THALAMUS		AMYGDALA & HIPPOCAMPUS		RAPHE NUCLEUS		LOCUS CERULEUS	

(© Tisserand Aromatherapy Limited 1988)

Nearly 80% of us with MS are first diagnosed because of changes in our vision. Vision is one of the most important senses we possess for retaining our independence. Probable loss of part, or all of our vision, is one of the most frightening experiences. Why does vision loss occur so frequently?

The eye or optic nerve is a part of the brain and spinal cord, (i.e. central nervous system). As such, it too, is susceptible to our errant white blood cells attacking, or chewing away on the myelin, the protective covering insulating our nerves. When this occurs, the body responds to the free radicals and cytokines with inflammation, the body's healing solution. Inflammation (like a sprained ankle) means swelling, heat, redness and pain (or loss of function). Swelling has a devastating effect on the optic nerve, because the optic nerve travels through a narrow aperture or hole in our bony skull. A small amount of swelling can temporarily reduce or minimize vision from that eye. Also, the shooting pain that some of us experience may be a secondary symptom of this inflammation.

During this stage of acute inflammation in MS, corticosteroids are often used by our physician. Other options include regular emu oil capsules, regular or periodic boost of glutathione enhancement, (with a whey protein isolate as discussed in Chapter 11) and the boosting of omega-3's from flax and/or fish oils. In addition, omega-3 fatty acids enhance tear production – especially important for some of us with Sjogren's Syndrome (dry eyes and dry mouth) or for people who wear contact lenses or who are considering corneal surgery.

Improved nutrition can protect and enhance our vision as we age. A diet high in natural antioxidants is the foundation for eye health. Specific supplements providing omega-3 fatty acids, lutein (minimum 2g per day) and bonded or bioactive cysteine (See Chapter 11 on Glutathione for details), are especially important. These supplements can slow down, even reverse, early cataracts and reduce our risk of macular degeneration and other eye problems (i.e. glaucoma).

In addition, success in one part of our brain and spinal cord (CNS) provokes similar improved well-being in other areas of the CNS. We too often forget that all of our body is linked with blood circulation, nerves, lymph flow and hormones. This is why improvement in one region, organ or organ system usually transfers benefits to others. An obvious link to vision is hearing. We know by raising glutathione in the inner ear, we can often improve our sense of hearing. Similarly, this same boost of GSH unfolds cataract crystals! As mentioned in Chapter 18, Walking, Balance and Nerve Pathway Retraining, people with MS become very eye dependent. Now we can look after our vision better, as well!

Finally, please refer to the vitamin/mineral chapter and the measurement of 18 carotenoids in skin with the biophotonic scanner technology. Some very important carotenoids, which are measurable with this device, and that are key in vision are beta-carotene, zeaxanthin and lutein. Therefore, in your health journey, consider having your skin carotenoid score done by this machine. It provides an objective measure which is linked to overall body health.

Proprioception is another sense I would like to highlight. Proprioception refers to knowing where our body parts, arms, legs, and trunk are relative to one another. Most of us with MS become hugely dependent on our eyes to compensate for loss of proprioception. Our neurologists examine us and use two tests for proprioception. One is the Romberg test. This is done standing with feet together and arms outstretched in front, palms up. We then close our eyes. Healthy individuals maintain their balance. Those with loss of proprioception lose their balance. For more than six years, I tended to fall on my butt. After "retraining" or recruiting back-up miniature motor nerve (gamma) pathways, I am pretty stable, even with my eyes closed. The second of these tests involves reaching from finger to nose and the neurologist's hand, quickly and repeatedly. I was awful at this but am much better, now. Similarly, my eye-hand co-ordination, which relies on vision and proprioception, is better. Once again, I can enjoy table tennis and swatting houseflies reasonably well!

Touch is a well-recognized sense as well. When my MS was at is worst, I needed to check the temperature of my shower water with my shoulder. Similarly, I cannot determine the coldness in my hands and feet until they actually turn white and start to hurt. My loss of light touch has progressed to covering my entire body. I am still looking for ways to remedy or "retrain" this challenge. Please note Jeannette Hughes' inspirational story as follows. You will see why "hope springs eternal" and how the possibility of change exists for us all.

Peaks and Valleys of My Journey
By JEANNETTE HUGHES

At 32 years of age, with five children under 10, I was diagnosed with multiple sclerosis. (I had my first attack eight years earlier, in 1963, but the small prairie hospital where I was treated failed to recognize the MS symptoms.) I have managed to keep myself going and accomplish a great deal despite all odds.

In 2004, I am a widow, working usually 14- to 16-hour days as a Sidney town councillor, and also an extremely active participant in many other aspects of the community. Although I have never said my life as a person with MS has been easy – far from it - I usually dwell on the peaks rather than the valleys.

During the first 10 years after I received the fateful news of my chronic illness, I experienced a significant attack requiring hospitalization every year. Severe loss of vision several times, numbness to the point that I had no feeling in my body from my neck down, and then a severe drug reaction disabled me further. Following one attack, I could not even write my name for six months and could not drive for 48 months although I later got behind an automobile wheel again for several years and, more recently, became so proficient on a scooter that I produced a video and wrote a pamphlet on scooter safety. I also wrestled with severe depression, partly because I had little moral support from a family who had trouble accepting my health situation. Rest, antidepressants and steroids were not the answer.

Trying to find answers for myself during this «dark decade,» I met several people with MS and started the first MS support group in the area of Vancouver Island where I then lived - which still is going strong after 30 years. Through the group, I found the courage to get back on my feet after every major attack, survive five teenagers, go to university, change my career from nursing to research and writing for the provincial Ministry of Health, divorce and live on my own for three years. I subsequently co-authored one book and authored another, prepared various pamphlets and guides, and wrote published articles about self-motivation and strategies for coping with adversity. In addition, I remarried, travelled and changed careers again . . . and even did some television production and became something of an expert in universal design.

The list of alternative therapies I have tried is so long I will mention only a few: pool therapy (swimming and water exercise), hot tub exercise, working with a trainer at the Body Barn Gym in Sidney (much more fun than a PT at the MS clinic), journal-writing, meditation (TM), visualization, dance therapy and laser acupuncture (which cured seven years of severe back pain). As well, I have experimented with various supplements.

Part of my survival strategies have been, resisting medical suggestions to go on drug trials, take pain killers, "just rest," use a back brace, and take steroids and numerous other drugs. Keeping an open positive mind and gaining control over my MS has allowed me to live an active fulfilled life. Of the supplements I have tried, the most dramatic results have been from the whey protein isolate (see Chapter 11).

More than 15 years ago, while cutting back my juniper bushes, my legs became severely scratched and bleeding, as I had no feeling in them. After six months on a particular whey protein isolate providing bioactive cysteine, one day an ant ran up my leg and I felt every tiny footprint. I realized that after all those years I was regaining feeling in my legs.

The foregoing is just a glimpse of my life, which has been enhanced in the past few years through the caring and constructive influence of Dr. William Code. It is a privilege to have this opportunity to thank him in print.

Chapter 17

Sexuality And Bladder Issues

The changes that take place in our bodies, secondary to MS, are quite varied. Some of the earliest changes may often involve the bladder and perineal/genital area. Once it is determined that we have MS, many of us can look back on the changes in our bladder patterns as being an often ongoing, persistent problem, that we had tried to explain to ourselves in some other way. I recall voiding troubles, particularly while standing, for 10-15 years prior to diagnosis. I falsely assumed that I must have had an early prostate partial blockage of the bladder outflow tract. My adaptation: I sat down to empty my bladder. Hesitancy in starting voiding is common in MS.

The most likely reason for early and/or persistent bladder changes is our anatomy. The nerve supply to the bladder and sexual organs has long and relatively small nerves running lengthwise from the brain to the lowest part of the spine. (The medical term is, 'cranio-sacral' outflow of the parasympathetic pathway.) These long, long small nerve tracts are quite likely to be more susceptible to early 'injury' by MS 'attacks' or demyelination.

Bladder symptoms for men and women include more frequent voidings (the emptying of all or part of the bladder). The incomplete emptying of the bladder creates a place in which bacteria can grow. This frequently results in bladder infections. This is especially likely in women, as the urethra (tube from bladder to outside) is particularly short (1-2 cms in women compared to10-15 cms in men). This short distance makes the female bladder especially vulnerable to bladder infections, particularly e.coli bacteria. This bacteria is a common component of our bowel tract and the feces from it. Hence, the importance, for women, of wiping front to back, and wearing cotton panties to prevent bladder infections. Women are also at risk for 'honeymoon cystitis', that is, bladder infection following frequent intercourse. 'Honeymoon cystitis' is believed to be due to the 'friction' or rubbing of intercourse which can inflame the urethral opening, making it more susceptible to bacterial infection. Emptying the bladder within 30-60 minutes of having intercourse can minimize these infections.

MS folks are more prone to bladder infection because the MS changes in the nerve supply causes incomplete emptying of the bladder. This residual urine is unfortunately a 'sitting duck' for infection. Urine contains warm water and protein, both of which are needed for rapid bacterial growth. In the past, residual urine could only be determined by in and out catheterization. Now a bladder ultrasound (similar to the one taken during pregnancy) is simple and non-invasive.

I developed a bladder infection due to preoperative catheterization prior to the repair of my badly fractured ankle in 1998. My flight from Vancouver – Toronto – Cleveland was a huge challenge. I was enroute to the International MS Symposium in a wheelchair, which precluded bladder emptying for a period of 6-8 hours. After a two-week trip involving many "cramps, urgencies and some sweats", a course of antibiotics quickly resolved the situation. I believed that my bladder problems were simply my MS getting worse.

This is an honest mistake, but points to the need for a high index of suspicion when dealing with bladder infections, especially in women with MS. Early diagnosis and treatment relieves many symptoms, but will also reduce your risk of the infection spreading 'upriver' to your kidneys. I believe regular, pure cranberry juice, dried cranberries or cranberry capsules are a useful assist for women with MS. Why? Because it

has been documented that the cranberry reduces the likelihood of e.coli bacteria 'implanting', or taking up residence
in the bladder wall. Both Denise and I recommend pure
cranberry juice, rather than the heavily sweetened cranberry
cocktail. If these simple steps are inadequate then visit your
physician for medical advice.

My relationship with a bright, well-trained urologist in
my city, Dr. Bill Nielsen, permitted one other useful nugget in
bladder troubles. Saw palmetto, by mouth, affects bladder
receptors. Until recently health care practitioners felt it
worked on slowing prostate enlargement and hence, only in
men. We now know a quality saw palmetto soothes some of
the key irritable bladder receptors. It is these irritated bladder
receptors which trigger those of us with MS to get up several
times a night. I suggest taking 15 ml or one tablespoon daily,
of a Canadian-researched, quality saw palmetto (in conjunction with damiana leaf, ginseng root, ginkgo biloba leaf and
muira puama wood) in liquid form. This limits me to one
bathroom wake-up call per night and, several women with
MS have also much improved their sleep pattern by using this
liquid, available without prescription. In fact, my Mexican
women friends tell me the same mixture minimizes the hot
flashes and symptoms of menopause!

Well, I have skirted the sexual changes of MS long
enough. The early sensory changes, particularly in the genital
area, often complicate sex in many ways. In women, the very
sensitive skin and mucosal surfaces of the vulva, labia and
vaginal entrance, or clitoris, can send mixed messages to
both partners. This hypersensitivity can actually be painful,
reducing the usual lubrication of foreplay and diminishing
coital pleasure and even eliminating it altogether. This is particularly troubling to a young couple – where one of the pair
has MS. The importance of caring, frank and patient discussion between the couple cannot be overstated.

The changes in our making love due to my MS,
occurred twenty years into our marriage. These changes are
usually earlier in women, as MS often begins in women in
the late teens, 20s & 30s.

Sexuality, and more importantly, intimacy, are key components of a lasting relationship. Relationships are a very important part of our mind, body, and spirit continuum. A healthy body, mind and spirit are key to our well-being, our recovery from, and our control of, our MS. Any resource, whether counseling, education, or even a weekend or longer away for the couple, is valuable.

Relationships are one of the most volatile issues for MS folks. When my health was spiraling downhill rapidly, I tried to push Denise away. I thought I was worthless and that I was on my way to the pit of despair or institutionalization. Even worse, I was worried that I would be a huge draw on our family's meager economic resources. But Denise was stubborn. She didn't budge. She was in our relationship for the long haul. This was incredibly important to me.

Over the last 5-6 years, our lovemaking has needed to adapt, and transcend the hectic lifestyle trials and tribulations of Denise's work and three children. The brain-erection connection has been virtually severed for me. This means local area touching and stroking is essential for erection to occur. Also, frequent feedback between the couple of what feels good, and what does not, is very important. This "brain connection" change means I can no longer tell whether I have an erection or not without seeing or hand checking. Similarly, I cannot usually tell if I am inside the vagina or not. Happily, the pleasures of touch and ejaculation are still in place. Similar situations happen to many people with MS, in different ways.

These changes are often aggravated by the 'mind numbing' fatigue of MS. The MS individual is often "too tired" to even be interested in sex. I believe "the invisible" fatigue is perhaps the most common and generally debilitating symptom of MS, as it occurs in 85% of us. Severe fatigue hampers MS folk's ability to adapt well to the change or loss of their senses, mobility or strength. Adaptation to change is a large component of what makes us human. For some years MS fatigue limited communication between Denise and I. Besides fatigue, I also experienced discomfort from minor touching.

This discomfort, which I labeled "naked nerve ending" impacted on feelings of intimacy, including sexual intimacy (even limiting skin to skin pleasurability). Reversal of fatigue has helped both of us, and our relationship, to progress forward to new levels of growth, trust and self-esteem.

Suggested Solutions:

1. Warm or even tepid baths, together with 'Epsom' salts, magnesium sulfate (bath salts) and aromatherapy. This time of relaxation, enhanced by aromatherapy, (i.e. lavender, will help intimacy to proceed. See Chapter 16 on the 5 senses for charts on Aromatherapy. (See Resources at back of book.)
2. Use of erotic oils for one or both partners. (Emu oil will lower pain hypersensitivity.) (See Resources at back of book.)
3. Time together away from our hectic world in peaceful, serene settings, best near nature!

Both # 1 and #2 above will tend to reduce the nerve irritability of MS and perhaps muscle spasms as well. The Joint Comfort product listed in the links at **www.emu.ca**, is often very helpful at reducing muscle pain and spasms, too.

Before completing this chapter, I believe it is important to include our suggestions for those with advanced MS – particularly bladder and sex. If MS progresses, catheterization may be required at some point. In my travels around North America, I have learned of a patented and FDA approved device that has a special valve, which helps pool, and intermittently flush out urine from the bladder. This more closely approximates the filling of a normal full bladder and then complete emptying of this greater volume. Similarly, it may reduce bladder infection with the "flushing" of this temporarily stored urine. Bladder spasms may be minimized as well. If the bladder can still fill somewhat, this could permit more normal sexual intercourse, by temporarily removing the catheter. One other option many of us do not know about is the supra pubic (above the pelvic bone) catheter. Ask your urologist if and when this would be a useful option.

Finally, many of the foregoing suggestions may reduce bladder infection, the bane of many MS folks' existence. Similarly, the enhanced cell-mediated immunity of our white blood cells, from increasing glutathione in the body, may reduce the frequency of antibiotics being required. See Chapter 11 on Glutathione (GSH) and its role in preventing infection. This is quite important, as many of us become either sensitized (allergic) or develop bacterial resistance to these antibiotics.

Chapter 18

Walking, Balance and Nerve Pathway Retraining

Loss of mobility, whether it is walking or using one's arms is frequently encountered in MS. The inability to walk has two contributing factors in my observation and experience. Often loss of balance or proprioception is one problem. Secondarily, loss of muscle strength aggravates the balance issue. Folks with MS will state one or the other, or both, as walking/mobility issues.

Let us start with what is perhaps the easiest to explain. In almost all cases, the muscles and the nerves that supply them are fine. We must remember, however, when a body tissue or pathway is unused it starts to fade or become ineffective. The motor nerve simply leaves the spinal cord and arrives at the muscle. But we need to understand that even though we started with some 250 muscles at birth, by our thirties we are down to 80, even as low as 50. Why such a difference? If you don't use it you lose it! This includes many of our less or almost never used muscles, like the ones that act as stabilizers for our standing and walking, and the fine-tuning muscles – such as the ones that pull our thighs together (adductors) or apart (abductors).

When any of our "walking" muscles are deprived of their nerve supply in our spinal cord or brain, that muscle use is diminished or even lost completely. Subsequently the body quickly learns a new "gait" or way of walking which is almost always abnormal and not efficient. It skews our walking, disturbs our balance and even affects some of our joints as well. I credit Meir Schneider, of California, for first introducing this to me, and credit some of my MS friends for reinforcing it. He was legally blind until 17 years of age before learning that he could recruit or retrain "back-up" motor nerve pathways. These are small eye muscles which control the eye's movement and "pairs" the two eyes' movement to avoid "double vision". Vision loss and double vision are common symptoms in MS and can often be minimized by "balancing" and "low light training of the eye". Meir was able to recover a considerable amount of his vision, which permitted a much more normal life, with improved, but not perfect vision.

The concept that Meir Schneider presented to us, first in Vancouver, and then later in Victoria, was that our body possesses the great feature of redundancy, or "back up" or "reserve" motor nerves. This means that the specialized motor nerve, which is so important in balance and eye-hand coordination (i.e. proprioception), also has backup nerves which can be recruited to perform the same function. Another example would be the common belief in regards to stroke recovery — whatever abilities a person gains back in the first two years following a stroke, these will be the only ones that he will <u>ever</u> gain back. But now we know that there are "spare" pathways that we can train. Also, the younger you are when you receive a brain injury, the better your chances are of a full recovery. This holds true for injuries to the spinal cord. In fact, you can remove one half of the brain of a newborn and they can develop completely normal!

New concepts about our brain and spinal cord continue to emerge. The 1990's was the "decade of the brain" in the research world and many contributions have shaken "old" ideas. For example, we only use an average of 10% of our brain during our lifetime. I always pause here briefly when speaking to an audience. Inevitably, one or a few people will smile. I then suggest that some of us are not even using that 10% yet! Are we saving it?! This concept is incredibly important to those of us with a brain illness such as MS or who have had a traumatic injury. We now know we should never give up or abandon hope of recovery.

Eva Marsh is the Canadian who wrote "Black Patent Shoes, Dancing with MS". She has been a person of great inspiration to me. She has been paralyzed a number of times with MS, but is still walking. Her education and research about the nervous system convinced her of this possibility. In fact, she had recovered from one of her bouts of almost total paralysis with the help of her two very young daughters. It wasn't easy, but it certainly was worth all the trouble, because the regaining of one's independence is invaluable. She describes her brain's MRI (Magnetic Resonance Imaging) as being a near white out. Apparently, when it is shown to neurologists, most of them ask how many years she has been in a wheelchair – but she is not!

Another point of note here is that your MRI is not necessarily consistent with your disability. What this means is a "bad" looking MRI, may be an MRI of a fairly normal, well-functioning individual with MS. The converse is also true. The biggest determinant of your outcome, or recovery, is the "dedication" or "effort" you put into this body, mind and spirit scenario.

The best example is people who have had a stroke, and have lost the ability to speak. Almost always, if they work at it, they can recover their speech. It may be as tough or even harder than the first time they learned to speak, but it can be done. They regain their speech, not because they have retrained the injured piece of brain, or that because this piece of brain has healed. Instead, what they have done is they have trained or "recruited" a completely new part of the brain.

A further useful piece of knowledge I received recently from a woman with her Masters in Speech Therapy, and her Masters in Voice (i.e. singing), was in regards to the speech problems of people who have MS. Her impression, with twenty years experience behind it, is that most folks with MS have reduced power and quality of speech due to inadequate breathing techniques. She has had great improvement from her own clients with Parkinson's disease. These methods of breathing can often be learned from voice/choir teachers in your own community. Better yet, a group or choir holds great benefits for the body, mind and spiritual growth and for new relationships as well. I find singing tenor in a choir a valuable component of my health and spiritual journey. Music, whether voice or an instrument, (i.e. keyboard, guitar or harp), are other great "recovery" or "nerve recruitment" methods. One other tip given to me by a wise physiotherapist specializing in MS is worth mentioning. If one of us with MS has a foot drop, but is not yet ready to accept a heel splint, there is another option. Buy a pair of lace-up boots, such as Roper boots or "granny" boots. The lace up support worked for me for the three years until I was able to retrain those muscles.

Balance is more challenging. Our awareness of where our body parts are enables us to stand, walk upright and all variations thereof. In MS we frequently lose this balance and become almost completely dependent on our visual cues. This is the basis of the Romberg test given to us by our physicians. In this we stand with our feet together, bare or stocking feet, hold our arms out in front of us and are asked to close our eyes. If we have MS, most often we will start to fall. Without our visual cues we cannot sense where our body parts are. In addition, those with reduced vision or "double" or blurred vision from MS are further challenged when standing or walking. Wisely, we should reach for a cane or walker to achieve a more stable, three pointed stance.

The above issues are further compounded by muscle weakness, whether from muscle disuse or Vitamin D deficiency (see vitamin D chapter). Again, our muscles are a "use it or lose it" proposition, hence the value of exercise.

How can we improve our proprioception, that is, awareness of where our body parts are? Happily these nerve pathways are miniature motor nerve pathways. This means that the information centers are spread across our muscles (i.e. gamma efferent fibers). When a muscle moves, these miniature motor nerve pathways send quick, tiny bits of information to the brain as the muscle contracts. This message to the brain is then coordinated with outgoing messages along nerves to smoothly move the muscle. Hence, if the major motor nerve pathway, let's call it #1 of 5, is interrupted in the spinal cord and/or brain, then the muscle does not move on command. Similarly, the miniature motor nerves that sense the position of the muscle are also interrupted. We perceive that we now have both less muscle strength and less awareness of where that muscle and hence body part is. These changes are why MS people often do badly on the Romberg Test (standing with eyes closed) and finger-nose pointing test. Our eyes take on the extra job of telling us where all our body parts are. As soon as our eyes are closed, we do poorly.

The perfect way to send much more mini-muscle traffic or pathway information to the brain is to exercise in front of the mirror. Move your arms slowly enough so your brain can retrain or recruit a group of new motor nerve position sense pathways. Here we use our eyes and muscle movement to retrain our position sense. An excellent lower limb recruitment method is to hold on to a chair, or something that is stable. While standing, lift one foot off the floor. Initially this is best done in front of a mirror, so that you can use your eyes to help. The more frequently we do this, moving our muscles through this range ourselves, or with an assistant, the more traffic we send to and from the brain and the quicker we will recruit new pathways. Similarly, even thinking about this adds more traffic. Now you can work at recruitment or retraining wherever and whenever you wish.

Before closing on such a positive note, I want to refer you to the chapter on fatigue, or energy management. If we are so tired, and we don't care about recruiting new pathways, it is unlikely to happen. The feelings of depression and hopelessness are issues that need to be dealt with. Please refer to the chapter on depression and ways to counteract same.

Finally, we all do better working in teams or pairs. As human beings, we all crave attention and support for our efforts. So, join your local yoga, exercise facility, MS support group or any similar group. Our local MS support group helped organize and subsidize yoga and tai chi for its members. Most MS support groups are part of MS Chapters which are affiliated with a region, state, province or National MS Society. Please look at the discussion on MS organizations because these have been a key component of my own health journey.

Each of us tends to identify with different heroes or we try to model ourselves after someone we trust and respect. To this end, we will now outline some people who have achieved a great deal despite the fact that they have MS.

Montel Williams is one of my favourite, physically active, MS people. His books are full of sensible, practical and achievable goals. Similarly, his talk show regularly displays empathy, trust and hope. Each of these is important in our own relationships and is necessary on our own roadway to recovery.

One of Montel's most recent books is "Body Change", The 21-Day Fitness Program for Changing Your Body ... and Changing Your Life!" This book was written in conjunction with his personal trainer, co-author, Wini Linguvic. The exercise routine incorporates aerobics, weight training, core and functional exercises to improve your balance, coordination, and strength. I cannot think of a better approach for any of us with MS, than the one taken by Montel Williams. Happily, this Body Change Program relies less on big complex machines and more on free weights, a bench and core exercises. The authors are accurate in calling their aerobics and weight training exercises straight forward. However, they also ask, "what about attitude? Each of us must personally grab onto a new motivation to improve ourselves. Montel & Wini hope that in reading about their efforts to surmount challenges on the road to keeping fit, or returning to fitness, that we will see whatever excuse we have for not training or not training harder, will be exposed for exactly what it is – an excuse.

Many of our family and friends want us to rest, to speed our recovery. Now, after eight years with MS, I believe "rest" is not the benefit we thought it was. Rest or "energy management" is a useful coping skill. However, physical use of our body, in a safe venue, is one of the best and most important components in our recovery. Certainly, a 21-day program may not fit with your capabilities at present. Why not a 42, 63 or 84-day program then? There is an incredible number of choices for us to follow and each one begins with a single step down that path.

After two years with no regular program, I have rejoined a fitness center. My current goal is to slow and, if possible, reverse the persistent osteopenia in my legs and the recently diagnosed first stage of osteoporosis of my spine. I, too, can forget my health journey is ongoing. My diet is pretty consistent, but so should be my physical activity. I am trying to be wiser by not beating myself up over this. I need to continue to like myself to facilitate my successful journey toward improved personal health and wellness.

A second individual's story that means a great deal to me is that of Meir Schneider, of San Francisco. I described earlier his considerable recovery of sight due to recruitment of back-up nerve pathways. When I first met him at the Vancouver Complementary Medicine seminar in 1997, he outlined his concepts. This excited me very much as a potential "recovery" program. At that time, I was relatively mobile, but dragged my right foot and was reasonably weak on my right side. He had us slowly rotate our neck, first one way and then another, and note how much flexibility we had. Then he asked us to do a series of exercises with our hands and feet (shoes off). He showed us the much improved flexibility in our neck which occurred as the result of using our hands and feet!

Denise noted a similar improvement as she still had residual neck stiffness after being kicked on the chin by a horse in 1995. Meir Schneider was able to convince most people in the room how interconnected our nervous and muscle systems are.

I learned more from him a year or so later at another conference hosted by the MS Society of B.C., Capital Region Chapter in Victoria. Since that time, I have read his books and watched his video. A young woman with significant MS who had walking problems, went to San Francisco to study under him. What she learned was a major part of her being able to walk normally again.

Many resources are available for us to start on our walking recovery or long-term maintenance. One of my favourite teachers is Brenda Adam-Smith. She is a physiotherapist with Feldenkrais training, who works for MS Canada, Capital Region Chapter, here in Victoria, B.C.

Her knowledge and study of new concepts, whether from the Alexander Technique, Meir Schneider's or others, suggests that the originators of these concepts is Dr. Moshe Feldenkrais, D. Sc. (1904-1984). I would like to tell you part of Dr. Feldenkrais' story as a tribute to his incredible contribution to those of us with MS or other CNS injuries (including stroke, cerebral palsy or back pain), muscle injuries or illnesses.

To begin this wonderful story, I will refer you to two books written by Feldenkrais students. The first is "Awareness Heals – The Feldenkrais method for Dynamic Health": by Steve Shafarman. The second book is "Relaxercise, The Easy New Way to Health & Fitness" by David Zemach-Bersin, Kaethe Zemach-Bersin and Mark Reese. Both of these are excellent and it is where I learned most of the Feldenkrais story. The original book by Moshe Feldenkrais is "Awareness Through Movement" (Harper & Row, 1972). In simple, concrete terms, the Feldenkrais Method (FM) eliminates any division between body and mind. With the FM you can begin to live in ways that minimize or eliminate many problems. Steve Shafarman's book uses simple, common movements: bending, turning, leaning, breathing, sitting and walking.

The discovery of the Feldenkrais Method had a fascinating background. Moshe Feldenkrais was born in the

Ukraine in 1904 and left home at the age of 14 to travel to Palestine mostly by foot. As a young man he studied in Tel Aviv, worked as a tutor, labourer and surveyor. He loved sports, particularly soccer, a game in which he severely injured the ligaments and cartilage of his left knee. In 1928, he moved to Paris to study physics, math, mechanical and electrical engineering. He went on to be Joliot-Courier's (winner of 1935 Nobel Prize in Chemistry) principal assistant. While in Paris, he met Jigors Kano, the developer of modern judo, and became one of the first Europeans to earn a black belt in judo.

In 1940, Moshe Feldenkrais escaped the Nazis by reaching England. He worked for the British Admiralty during World War II, helping to develop sonar and submarine detection. His wife, Yona Rubenstein, was a pediatrician. Throughout those years in his wife's office, he became very interested in human development, in children's movement, and especially the movement of babies.

A bus accident aggravated his soccer knee injury. Surgeons offered only a 50% chance of recovery, so he went his own way. In pursuit of a better answer, he studied everything that was then known about health and healing. This included anatomy and physiology, neuro-physiology, exercise and movement therapies, psychotherapy and spiritual practices, yoga, hypnosis and acupuncture.

Feldenkrais, despite his refusal of surgery, succeeded in learning to walk again, and even resumed his judo. His months of careful minimal movements with disciplined self-observation, enabled him to reawaken and refine young children's learning processes to move and function. In summary, he found the key to healing was to become more "aware" of what one is doing.

He went on to regain full movement of his knee. Furthermore, he helped a friend and fellow scientist to similarly recover from severe, chronic back pain.

Denise and I now understand, especially from our personal trainer here in Duncan, Judy Lamontagne, the ability of our body to adapt, and take "shortcuts" or "easy solutions".

This occurs frequently in weight training, and Judy and her staff ensure that the desired maneuver is always consistent. This is especially critical in our walking and gait.

When the body loses a muscle or group thereof, due to MS, it usually makes do, or substitutes a movement to "replace" the other. Unfortunately, this often complicates our gait and sometimes reduces our strength, joint mobility and mobility options. Then, when we recruit new nerve pathways, through our focus and effort, the muscle may recover, but our gait does not. What I mean is the body still uses the "shortcut" it had adapted to, and ignores the recovery of normal gait. It is up to us to seek out a knowledgeable trainer, physiotherapist, Feldenkrais-trained individual or a specialist like Meir Schneider to permit normal gait and walking again.

In late 1998, the retraining of my muscles was extremely difficult after a complex ankle fracture and orthopedic surgery, which involved six months in a wheelchair, and then several weeks on arm crutches (see back cover of this book). I had to work at recovering almost all of my muscle strength and then normalize my gait. My greatest fear was not being able to walk again. Loss of gait or walking is quite common in people with progressive MS, and particularly so after a major trauma and after months of not using our legs. We all know how much muscle disappears in 3-4 weeks, let alone 5-6 months. Certainly my decent recovery and that of several of my MS friends has made me passionate for hope for more MS people. I believe almost all of us can do this – the sooner the better. All recovery needs to get started and only we can take on this challenge ourselves. Many good coaches surround us, if we touch base with our local MS Society's suggested resources.

For any of us with MS who are still quite mobile, I suggest you do a modest amount of "training" to keep it that way. Yoga, Chi Gong and especially Tai Chi come to mind. I started Tai Chi some months ago and firmly believe that if someone learns the series of movement and focuses on them for one to two hours a week, the results will be awesome. Tai Chi is a set of moves that become almost reflex, after some 1,000 correct repetitions. This recruits and trains many of our "back-up" and "dormant" spinal and brain pathways. Subsequently, if MS injures some of our original pathways, we will have ready and waiting, these other Tai Chi-trained pathways. Doesn't that make you feel you are in control of your own destiny? It should!

Chapter 19

Continuing the Journey

The foregoing chapters are our attempt at helping you with a roadmap toward health and wellness. Not all suggestions will apply to you or work for you. However, I believe most of the suggestions will be helpful, and some of the suggestions will help you a great deal. Only you can determine this. For Denise and I, our education, work experience and crisis with illness have added to our wisdom. Our goal is to share this with you – in this book and through ongoing health teaching.

The first chapter outlined my early years of illness, 1996-2000. In this final chapter I will bring you up-to-date on my own journey and summarize a list of "Dr. Code's Choices for Chronic Illness".

Certainly, the first change or improvement on my road to recovery was reduced fatigue. Admittedly, this was a small baby step, but I became better at seeing and appreciating small changes. Not being quite as exhausted was the first improvement. I attributed this to the teaspoon of emu oil I was taking – in the hope that its anti-inflammatory effect would benefit me. Coupled with this was slightly longer ability to stand, before needing to sit down. However, I still dragged my right leg and could "trip" without a reason.

Somewhere, about April 1997, most of my light touch returned. I attributed this to intravenous chelation by my naturopath, after he determined from a urine and hair sample, that I had an excess of lead, a heavy metal. My clarity of thinking also improved. However, it took five more months for me to regain my hospital privileges.

The regaining of my hospital privilege required legal assistance and was coupled with my Dad's cancer, and in September 1997, his death. My anesthesia colleagues even required a psychiatric statement of my well-being and adequacy of mental health. This was particularly devastating to Denise in that all my depression and personal health issues had quickly traversed our small community. Yes, I was angry, too, perhaps more so with myself, for my sharing the personal matter of my depression with friends and colleagues (two of my three departmental members). However, I was nearly numb with frustration and primarily wanted to be able to restart my anesthesia career or "life". Finally, push came to shove, somewhere, and I started back to work on a temporary basis in late 1997.

My hand numbness returned after three successive Fridays back in the operating room. My family doctor advised against further anesthesia practice and I realized she was right, albeit, not permanently, just then. The hospital administration and my anesthesiology "friends and colleagues" nailed down the coffin some four weeks later. This was achieved with some careful and complicit manipulation of dates and paperwork on their part. This confirmed my decision to discontinue working, as I would have to start at the beginning as a new applicant for anesthesiology staff privileges – full time or nothing. I knew I was beat so I quit banging my head against the wall.

My next option was a civil suit against my anesthesiology colleagues and the hospital. Unfortunately, this would have had to be completely on my own nickel. The Canadian Medical Protective Association would have had to defend the practicing anesthesiology individual in this scenario. Sure, Denise and I were really angry and hurt. My family and I wanted to achieve fairness, restitution and even revenge. But, we were financially broke as well, and long, slow legal processes are very expensive. In addition, I might only achieve another chance to resume anaesthesiology practice.

My health may not have permitted success with another try. I finally said, "enough", and moved on from needing to resume my medical career, to the recognition that my health and my family were more important. This painful step was a critical turning point in my personal health journey. I hope it will permit you to make the correct decisions for yourself. Would I do it differently now, seven years later? Possibly. Could or can I? Probably not.

Personal crisis, whether physical, mental or emotional, can contribute to our health journey. Resolution of the crisis, often by letting go of our anger, and / or forgiveness, can resolve this crisis. The only one we can truly control is ourselves. Those around us are factors, which we can influence a little, but never control.

Despite the above insight, my touch in my hands has never returned. In fact, I have lost light touch on my entire body. Maybe, just maybe, it has improved on my left side in the past few months. I believe this is possible because several of my health choices will continue to reduce the toxins within me. These include lots of purified water, glutathione building blocks, organic and/or natural foods and an organic origin multivitamin/multi mineral. Coupled with these are exposure to clean air, water and environment, as much as possible.

Small steps of improvement occurred over the next four years. Emu oil, plenty of ground flax, rest, reduced stress and the life cycle on our small acreage were part of this gradual blunting of my super sensitivity to sound, motion and smell. I regained my balance. My migraine headaches became much less frequent when I gave up wheat, containing the subset of gluten, called gliadin. Personally, I suspect this may have reduced one of my MS triggers. To the list of foods to avoid, personally, I have added cheese, milk, yogurt, wine with sulfites (as preservatives), and scotch whiskey. I will occasionally cheat and have ice cream. Also, I still take four pouches of whey protein isolate daily. It has no casein or fatty acids in it, and therefore does not have the possible MS trigger in it called butyrophilin. This should reassure most of us who are in agreement with the important items to avoid in our diet relative to the Paleolithic diet.

The next major piece of the puzzle was my learning about this whey protein isolate as a useful building block for glutathione in every cell. As of late 2001, I started on a packet or envelope every day for three months. I noticed no difference. However, after speaking to research scientists in eastern Canada, I increased this to three packets per day. Their premise was that by the time I was diagnosed with a major neurodegenerative disease such as MS or Parkinson's, the glutathione in my body cells could be as low as 5% of normal.

Happily, within a month of being on three packages a day, my energy began to significantly improve. Within another 2-3 months, I felt I had enough energy to book in with a personal trainer to recover some of my strength, balance and coordination. Over four months I made steady progress, to both my surprise and everyone else's. My right leg limp almost disappeared. My muscle strength improved, and my need to sit down soon after standing almost disappeared. I could walk considerable distances! You can imagine my sense of well-being five years after losing most of these abilities. I wanted to talk about hope again with MS, rather than just endure the inevitable.

My pain and muscle spasms started to recede, until after six months on three packets a day, they were nearly gone. I had some slight improvement in mental clarity and cognitive ability, but only minimal. However, my hypersensitivity to smells, sounds and "bumps" on the road while in a car diminished a fair bit. My disappointment in my lack of cognitive ability was tempered somewhat, as I had already learned that cognitive impairment is only slightly linked to the degree of physical disability. My sense of touch has not improved but I can live with that.

By late 2002, I had found a short-term energy tonic which worked to enhance focus and concentration for several hours. By now, I had given up coffee, tea or cola drinks because they left me feeling jangled and shaky, plus they gave me diarrhea. Caffeinated products often cause flare-ups in those of us with irritable bowel syndrome. This herbal drink acutely raises your potassium and magnesium. It also contains, guarana, a slow 6-8 hour burn xanthine. It has similar effects to caffeine, but causes fewer high spikes and is more sustained.

Now, in late 2004 I am up to the toilet to void or empty my bladder once or twice a night. I have had half as many trips at night while on a high quality saw palmetto product, also containing damiana, ginseng and ginkgo biloba. It is now understood that saw palmetto calms many of our irritable bladder receptors. Hence, it is equally indicated in both men and women with MS. I still need to double void, i.e. two trips to empty my bladder more completely. If bladder infections, especially in women, are commonplace, refer to Chapter 17 – Sexuality and Bladder Issues for information. If an indwelling catheter is required, consider a valve unit to better simulate more normal bladder flushing, and to help prevent bladder spasms or infections. I hope to defer catheters as long as possible because they can cause low-grade infections, and the fever from infection seems to worsen MS symptoms.

The general heat sensitivity of our brain and spinal cord tissues is why so many of us with MS avoid sunlight. Avoiding bright sunlight costs us vitamin D and optimal melatonin production as mentioned previously. This awareness of injured brain vulnerability is also of concern in regards to the use of general anesthesia drugs. I suggest MS people consider spinal, epidural or regional anesthesia (freezing the nerves) whenever possible. In recent years anesthesiologists have also leaned in this direction. If fear of "being awake" is your issue, they have many other choices to transport you to "never, never land" temporarily. Please recall my two years in lab research on how general anesthetics has influenced my approach to this general anesthesia (G.A.) issue. Personal stories I have heard include a gerontologist asking six elderly Nobel Prize winners how long after a GA before they felt their brain worked normally again. They averaged six months in their replies. I believe caution in any brain illness or injury is prudent.

Issues involving my cognitive problems bear further comment as well. Firstly, I continue to improve, even if only slightly, a little at a time, month by month. I do not know if this is brain recovery, or improved adaptation or even recruitment of other parts of the brain. It may even be a composite of all three. I do know my creativity is slightly better, as is my patience. These compensate somewhat for the concrete linear clarity of problem solving I once enjoyed.

Of interest, I was asked by my disability insurance company to have an independent assessment done by an expert in MS at Scripps Clinic, LaJolla, California in 2002. My medical records, including my MRI preceded me. This very experienced neurologist was quite impressed with my degree of recovery. In noting this to me, he asked what I felt my toughest problem was – I replied, "Brain fog". He was having none of this and wanted a detailed explanation. I did my best to explain my lack of multi-tasking, my poor quality short-term memory and so on. He was not enamored with my ability to put this in scientific terms. Then he sent me for his pet or "favourite" test on cognitive function. This was a timed performance of addition and subtraction of the second or third last number. I did fair at the gentle speed, abysmally at the normal speed, and even worse at a moderately faster speed. He seemed completely able to accept my explanation once he saw the objective data.

Now, many of you would say "Aren't they going to give me a similar second chance for a second opinion?" My own neurologist, Dr. Don Paty, here in Canada, had already told me it was quite unusual to fly someone to an expert in another country. Dr. Paty, as mentioned in my dedication to him in the front of this book, was one of a handful of MS experts on the planet. You could also ask, was I at my best? Well, no, I do not want to be "at my best" but more typically should be at my worst when being assessed. Neither you nor I have any control of our best and worst days. Hence, when assessed or completing paperwork we need to record our worst-case scenarios. Why? – because almost every disability is seen as static or fixed. Woe to you if you take the Pollyanna or best possible day approach. Certainly, denial is your option, but if your health care practitioner and disability assessor is going to be able to fairly assess you, this is the only recommendation I can give you.

An interesting parallel to this is your own history of previous MS attacks recalled from your memory. These attacks mean much less than those episodes documented by a physician at the time. Please remember that. This advice may help you a great deal in the challenging financial journey you are on with this Multiple Sclerosis (or other chronic illness) diagnosis. My experienced family physician tried to end on an optimistic note as to my potential recovery. The agencies reviewing your case will always hook on to this "reduced disability" and go there, **not** to where you are.

One of my recovery puzzle pieces did not fall into place until the last half of 2004. This is when Denise started, with due diligence, working with the biophotonic scanner noted in the chapter on antioxidants. Prior to this I had used the multivitamin/multimineral recommended by Centre for Science in the Public Interest. Now, if people are able to afford it, or want to learn how they can "earn" it, go to the resources section. This further piece of the puzzle has made a difference in both of these 51-year-old folks (Denise and I)! In addition, this company sources almost all their components organically.

For the ultimate short summary you will note the "Dr. Code's Choices for Chronic Illness". You can send for a copy, with a stamped, self-addressed envelope, or get it online at **www.emu.ca** (see Resources). As new and different information emerges, Denise and I expect to learn more while on our journey to wellness. Your journey is in your hands and even small steps can make a difference. Our goal is to provide a roadmap of what we recommend. You, too, are an individual and you can and should fine-tune it yourself. Work with your health care practitioners as they still have access to any surgical or pharmaceutical solutions available. Make them your coaches, not dictators. You are in control of your MS, chronic illness, and your life! Good luck

To purchase Dr. Code's latest book, "Who's in Control of Your MS? Pieces of The MS Recovery Puzzle", or for a copy of Dr. Code's Corner Newsletter, go to the Resources section at the back of this book.

Dr. Code's 10 Choices for Chronic Illness

1. **Daily Omega-3 fat intake** – 2 Tablespoons of freshly ground flax will supply alpha-linolenic acid (omega-3 fat) and lignans. Lignans decrease the incidence of heart attack, stroke, breast and colon cancer. A daily fish oil supplement containing both fish and krill oils is the best way to boost the omega-3 fat, especially DHA needed for brain health.

2. ***4000 IU of Vitamin D daily*** – This will optimize the immune system, and reduce cancer and autoimmune conditions. This will also help your body absorb more calcium – important for preventing osteoporosis.

3. ***One multivitamin/multimineral supplement daily*** – Make sure it contains folic acid, B6 and B12. Tablets should disintegrate in water within two to four hours.

4. ***Use of digestive enzymes (4each meal) and daily probiotics*** – This will help enhance digestion and nutrient absorption.

5. ***1000 mg elemental calcium*** and ***500 mg magnesium daily*** – This will help maintain bone health.

6. **Use only healthy fats and oils** (i.e., quality olive oil) and butter or coconut oil for cooking at higher heats. ***Avoid trans fats***. These are hydrogenated vegetable oils found commonly in baked goods and deep-fried foods. Read food labels. This will greatly reduce your risk of heart attack and stroke.

7. ***Undenatured whey protein isolate in sealed packet form*** – This optimized the immune system, provides antioxidant benefits, and helps in detoxification. Quantity will depend on individual health needs.

8. ***Emu oil daily*** – Four to five gel caps will improve energy and mental focus, and will often thicken hair. Emu oil is an anti-inflammatory (topical and internal); very useful for pain relief and wound healing.

9. ***Avoid foods to which you are sensitive*** – This may include wheat gluten (gliadin) and sources of dairy casein (e.g., cheese, milk, yogurt).

10. ***Enjoy regular daily exercise and...keep hydrated*** – Find some form of physical activity you enjoy (e.g., walking, swimming, cycling, weights, Yoga, Tai Chi, pilates), preferably with a cardio-respiratory component. And, do drink 8-10 glasses of purified water daily.

Glossary

absorb – (nutrition) to draw nutrients from the gastrointestinal tract into the bloodstream.

acquired immune deficiency syndrome (AIDS) – a deficiency in the immune system due to infection by the human immunodeficiency virus (HIV).

ADHD – Attention Deficiency Hyperactivity Disorder: a condition characterized by inability to concentrate, focus or sit still. Often medicated with *Ritalin*. Has been linked to a deficiency in omega-3 fatty acids.

aerobic exercise – any physical activity that makes the heart and lungs work harder to meet the muscles need for oxygen.

albumin – a major protein found in blood serum.

allergy – an inappropriate immune response to a non-pathogen.

alveoli – tiny air sacs of the lungs where carbon dioxide leaves the blood and oxygen is taken on by the blood.

Alzheimer's– prolonged free radicals degenerative disorder.

amino acids – organic chemical compounds from which all proteins are made.

anaerobic exercise – oxygen is used by the muscles faster than it can be supplied by the bloodstream.

anaesthesiologist – a doctor of medicine graduate who studies five years to specialize in caring for people during surgery, intensive care and pain management.

anaphylaxis – a sudden and rapid swelling of the body, especially breathing and airway. Usually an allergic response.

anemia – low hemoglobin (red blood cell) count.

anthocyanins – any of several water-soluble nitrogenous pigments which contribute to the red, blue, or violet colors in some plants (e.g., cherries, grapes, plums). Powerful antioxidants.

atherosclerotic plaque – fatty or waxy substance that builds up in arteries leading to arteriosclerosis (hardening of the arteries).

antigen – substance foreign to the body that triggers an immune response.

antigen response – immune systems response to an antigen.

anti-inflammatory – drug or compound that reduces the symptoms of inflammation.

antioxidant – a substance that neutralizes destructive free radicals or prevents oxidation; some are manufactured by the body, others are derived from foods.

arthritis – inflammation of joints characterized by pain, heat, redness, swelling and stiffness, sometimes leading to deformation of the joint.

asthma – recurrent bouts of breathlessness of varying severity due to constriction of the small airways.

autoimmune disease – dysfunctional immune response to healthy processes; disorder caused by inappropriate immune response to one's own tissue.

B. bifidus – a beneficial bacteria that lives in the gut.

bad fats (damaging) – *trans* (hydrogenated modified) dietary fats, especially when consumed in excess.

beta carotene – a precursor of vitamin A found in carrots, tomatoes, etc., and converted in the body to vitamin A.

bioactivity – the initiation of specific metabolic activity by a nutrient or other compound.

bioavailability – the amount of a biological substance available for a bodily process.

biochemical – chemical compounds produced by or interacting with the body.

blood sugar – the amount of glucose in the blood.

cancer – a group of diseases characterized by unrestricted growth of cells in a tissue or a specific organ.

candida – thrush or moniliasis; a fungal infection.

carcinogen – cancer-causing agent.

carotenoid – yellow or red pigments such as carotenes

found widely in plants and animals.

carrier oils –used in topical skin application and/or aromatherapy.

casein – milk protein; one of the proteins in milk.

cataract – loss of transparency of the lens of the eye due to changes in the delicate protein fibres within the lens.

cell – basic structural element of the body; trillions in number and highly differentiated in function.

cerebro-spinal fluid – a clear, watery liquid that surrounds and infuses the brain and the central canal of the spinal cord.

chelation – the attachment of toxins present in the body to organic compounds, allowing their excretion and resulting in diminished toxicity.

chelators – organic compounds that attract and stick to metal molecules.

cholesterol – an important fatty constituent of body cells; a player in the formation of hormones and the transport of fats to various parts of the body; HDL (good) cholesterol protects against arterial disease; LDL (bad) cholesterol promotes arterial disease.

chronic – of long duration; with diminished likelihood of cure.

chronic inflammatory change – persistent inflammation and its biochemical changes.

chronic inflammatory disease – persistent diseases characterized by inflammation, such as rheumatoid arthritis.

cis fatty acid – a fatty acid configuration where the hydrogen atoms of the carbon atoms involved in the double bond are on the same side of the molecule, causing the molecule to bend or kink.

cold pressed – oils extracted from seeds or nuts without the use of hexane, and done at low temperatures.

colitis – general inflammation of the bowel.

collagen – the main protein substance of the body; responsible for the form and shape of most tissues (except bone and cartilage).

colon – the major part of the large intestine.

comedogenic (non-comedogenic) – acne causing (non-acne causing).

complementary medicine – the combined application of conventional and alternative health practices.

complex carbohydrate – sugar molecules strung together to form longer, more complex chains. Complex carbohydrates include starch and fiber.

constipation – infrequent and difficult passing of hard feces.

cosmeceutical – a cross between a "cosmetic" and a "pharmaceutical" – a cosmetic product that is expected to have some therapeutic or active beneficial component(s).

cysteine – a sulfur-containing amino acid; scarcest of the three constituents of GSH.

cystic fibrosis – mucoviscidosis; an inherited, congenital disease characterized by chronic lung infection and poor absorption of nutrients.

degenerative disease – physical and/or chemical changes in cells, tissues or organs leading to progressive impairment of both structure and function.

delta-5-desaturase – an enzyme in the human body that converts components of fatty acids to "bad" eicosanoids. This enzyme is not present in the skin.

dementia – a general decline of mental functioning.

depression – feelings of sadness, hopelessness, pessimism, loss of interest in life and diminished emotional well-being.

dermatitis – any mild or moderate inflammation of the skin causing rash and/or itchiness.

dermis – the thick layer of living tissue below the epidermis (skin).

detoxifier – any substance that neutralizes toxins, pollutants and carcinogens.

desensitize – slowly and gradually reduce response, e.g., allergy to bee stings; or fear of heights.

diarrhea – increased fluidity and frequency of bowel movements; a symptom of underlying disease.

disease – an unhealthy condition of the body or mind; illness, sickness.

distress – stress beyond the body's ability to respond favorably.

diverticuli – tiny pouch-like sacs that develop in the colon, becoming inflamed when matter becomes lodged in them.

dopamine – a neurotransmitter found in the brain.

duodenum – first part of small intestine, after the stomach.

dysfunction – abnormal activity; inability to function.

eclampsia – a rare, very serious condition of late pregnancy causing seizures and coma.

eczema – inflammation of the skin.

eicosanoids – hormone-like substances that regulate blood pressure, clotting, immune response, inflammation response and other body functions; formed from omega-6 and omega-3 fatty acids.

emollient – a substance that softens tissues, especially the skin and mucous membranes.

emu oil – contains Omega-3 and 6 essential fatty acids along with an anti-inflammatory pigment, probably a carotenoid. Can be used as a therapeutic carrier oil.

emulsify – to mix a liquid into another liquid, making a suspension that has globules of fat.

emulsion – a mix of two liquids, made so that small droplets are formed, as oil and water.

endogenous antioxidants – antioxidants produced within the body.

endorphins – the body's own natural pain killers.

enzyme – any protein that promotes or regulates a specific chemical reaction in the body.

Epstein-Barr virus – a DNA herpes virus which causes infectious mononucleosis.

essential amino acids – amino acids that must be obtained from dietary sources and cannot be manufactured by the body; arginine, histidine, isoleucine, leucine, lysine, methionine, phenylalanine, threonine, tryptophan and valine.

essential fatty acids – (**EFAs**) several varieties of fatty acids that must be eaten because the body cannot manufacture them. Essential to brain function, manufacture of enzymes and for the integrity of the cell wall.

fat – nutrient providing the body with its most concentrated form of energy; a solid or liquid oil of vegetable or animal origin.

fiber – the indigestible portion of the diet consisting of various plant cell-wall materials, that passes through the body largely unchanged.

fiber foods – foods containing indigestible plant material that holds water and adds bulk to the feces, aiding normal bowel function.

fibroblasts – cells producing collagen fibers in connective tissue of the body.

flavonoids – a variety of crystalline compounds found in plants; some are powerful antioxidants.

flu (influenza) – contagious virus infection causing fever, severe aching, weakness and coughing.

free radicals – oxyradical; a highly reactive molecule with one or more unpaired electrons; free radical destruction is implicated in a wide variety of diseases.

GABA – gamma-aminobutyric acid; a neurotransmitter.

gingivitis – inflammation or infection of the gums accompanied by any combination of pain, swelling, and bleeding.

glaucoma – optic nerve fiber destruction and gradual loss of vision caused by increased fluid pressure within the eye.

glucose – a simple sugar containing six carbon atoms, which is an important energy source.

glutamine – a crystalline amino acid found in plant and animal protein.

glutathione – GSH; a crystalline, water-soluble tripeptide composed of glutamic acid (glutamate), cysteine and glycine.

glutathione peroxidase – a critically important antioxidant enzyme.

glycine – an amino acid and neurotransmitter.

GSH – glutathione; multifunctional tripeptide composed of glutamate, cysteine and lysine.

GSH peroxidase – an enzyme of glutathione critical as an antioxidant, especially against lipid peroxidation.

gut – stomach and intestines.

hair follicles – small pits in the epidermis that grow individual hairs.

half-life – period required by the body to eliminate or metabolize a substance to 50% levels.

hexane – a chemical used to extract oil from seeds and nuts.

HDL cholesterol – high density lipoprotein; a component of blood that carries cholesterol but protects against arteriosclerosis; also known as "good cholesterol".

helicobacter pylori – H. pylori; one of a large family of related bacteria that live in the stomachs of most vertebrates.

hemoglobin – a complex protein within red blood cells responsible for carrying oxygen to all other cells.

high blood pressure – hypertension; abnormally high blood pressure.

high carbohydrate, low fat diet – a diet that, because it is low in fat, is supposed to be good for weight loss.

homocysteine – a peptide that either promotes arteriosclerosis or is found in conjunction with arteriosclerosis; a potential risk factor for hardening of the arteries; a substance that is converted from methionine, an amino acid.

hormone – a chemical released by an endocrine gland into the bloodstream that affects remote tissues and other hormones in specific ways.

human immunodeficiency virus – HIV; the virus that leads to AIDS.

hydrogenation – the addition of hydrogen to an edible oil to convert it into a trans fat and saturated fat, usually solid at room temperature.

hypercholesterolemia – a condition characterized by an excess of cholesterol in the bloodstream.

hyperlipidemias – any condition characterized by an excess of fats in the bloodstream.

hyperthyroidism – overactivity of the thyroid gland, resulting in a rapid heartbeat and an increased rate of metabolism.

hypothyroidism – decreased activity of the thyroid gland.

idiopathic – of unknown cause.

immune response – activation of the immune system; ability of the body to protect against microbes, toxins, free radicals and other threats.

immune system – a system of cells and proteins that protect the body from potential harm.

incidence – frequency; a statistical measure.

indigestion – difficulty in digesting food; pain or discomfort caused by this.

inflammation – redness, swelling, heat and pain in a tissue due to injury or infection.

inflammatory bowel disease – chronic intestinal inflammation, including ulcerative colitis and Crohn's disease.

innocuous – harmless, non-toxic.

insomnia – inability to sleep.

insulin – a polypeptide hormone produced in the pancreas by the islets of Langerhans, which regulates the amount on glucose in the blood, and the lack of which causes diabetes.

intestines – the principal part of the gastrointestinal tract, reaching from the exit of the stomach to the anus.

intravenous – within the blood circulation.

ischemia – blood starvation; oxygen deprivation resulting from inhibited blood flow.

Islets (or Islands) of Langerhans – small parts or globules of special cells (millions of them) within the pancreas. These islets secrete insulin and glucagons.

lactalbumin – a specific type of whey protein.

lactic acid – a carboxylic acid formed in the muscle tissues from glucose and glycogen during strenuous exercise.

lactose – milk sugar.

lactose-intolerance – inability to digest lactose accompanied by nausea, cramps and diarrhea.

lactobacillus acidophilus – a good bacteria present in the gut.

LDL cholesterol – low density lipoprotein (bad) cholesterol associated with increased risk of arteriosclerosis.

lesion – pathological area of tissue.

life process – a stage of life such as growth, puberty and menopause.

lipids – fatty substances.

liver – large, lobed, glandular organ in the abdomen, responsible for metabolizing fats, detoxifying and neutralizing foreign and toxic substances.

Lou Gehrig's disease – ALS; amyotrophic lateral sclerosis; a rare, fatal, progressive, degenerative autoimmune disease of the nervous system that usually begins in middle age; characterized by increasing muscular weakness.

lupus – a chronic autoimmune disease causing inflammation of connective tissue.

lycopene – a carotenoid antioxidant found in brightly-coloured vegetables and fruits.

lymphocyte – a type of white blood cell crucial to the adaptive part of the immune system and made in the lymph nodes, bone marrow, and thymus gland; lymphocytes identify and 'remember' invading disease organisms.

melatonin – a hormone produced in the body and which helps us sleep.

membrane – a layer of usually very thin tissue that covers a bodily surface or forms some sort of barrier.

metabolism – all chemical processes taking place in the body; catabolic metabolism breaks down complex substances into simpler ones; anabolic metabolism manufactures complex substances from simple building blocks; the life process of cell, which takes place in the mitochondria of the cell.

metabolize – to convert foods and other biochemicals into living bodily processes.

methionine – a thiol amino acid (sulphur containing).

migraine – an intermittent disorder of uncertain origin provoking vision disturbances, nausea and severe, long-lasting headaches.

mitochondria – energy-generating component of cells.

modulate – to adjust in a controlled manner.

modulation – changing the amount of a substance; regulation of levels.

monosaccharides – a sugar that cannot be hydrolyzed to simpler carbohydrates of smaller carbon content. Glucose and fructose are examples.

monounsaturated fatty acids – fatty acids whose molecules contain one double bond in its carbon chain (contains one point of unsaturation).

mortality – death rate statistic.

motility – description of movement, e.g., food along intestinal tract.

multifactorial – having several causes or effects.

multiple sclerosis – a progressive, unpredictable disease of the nervous system of auto-immune cause.

muscle – tissue consisting of elongated cells (muscle fibers) containing fibrils that are highly contractile.

mycoplasma – types of microorganism without cell walls that are intermediate between viruses and bacteria and are mostly parasitic.

myelin – fatty insulating sheath enclosing nerve fibers.

natural product – a substance found in nature as opposed to a pharmaceutical product; also applied to substances found in nature but rendered to unnatural levels of concentration or purity.

naturopath – one who practices alternative medicine using a non-pharmaceutical approach.

negative feedback inhibition – balancing factor in which increased levels of a biochemical substance cause its continued secretion to slow down or stop.

nerve impulses – messages passed between the brain and various parts of the body through the nerves.

neural plaque formation – build-up of protein deposits in brain tissue and spinal cord.

neurodegenerative disorder – any progressive disease of the nervous system caused by physical and/or chemical changes of the brain and its chemical balance.

neurological – having to do with the brain and/or nervous system.

neuron – cell of the brain and nervous system.

neuropathy – disease, damage or inflammation of peripheral nerves.

neurotransmitter – a chemical released from nerve endings that transmits information among neurons.

neutralize – to render ineffective; antioxidant donation of an electron to stabilize electrical charge.

non-food – any "food" that contains no life energy – few vitamins, minerals, fiber or anything beneficial to sustain health; usually processed and packaged.

nutriceuticals – new term that describes therapies based on or including foods and food supplements.

nutritionist – health practitioner specializing in nutrition, alimentation and absorption.

oral antioxidant supplements – concentrated food-like substances that help the body neutralize free radicals.

organic compounds – all compounds containing carbon, except carbon oxides, carbon sulfides and metal carbonates.

osteoporosis – loss of protein matrix tissue from bone causing it to become brittle and to lose structural integrity.

over-training syndrome – negative effects on the body of excessive amounts or intensity of exercise.

oxidation – the normal process by which matter is metabolized to energy using oxygen.

oxidative stress – cellular and tissue damage resulting from oxidation and leading to bodily disorders. oxidized glutathione – GSSG; paired glutathione molecules that have neutralized free radicals by absorbing two negatively charged ions.

oxyradical – free radical; a molecule that through the natural process of oxidation is deprived of an electron and rendered toxic.

pancreas – a digestive organ/gland in the body which manufactures digestive enzymes as well as insulin and glucagons, hormones vital to control of blood sugar levels in the body.

panic attack – a period of acute anxiety, sometimes focused on the fear of death or loss of reason.

paranoia – a delusion that certain persons or events are especially connected to oneself.

Parkinson's disease – shaking palsy; a neurological disorder characterized by muscular tremors, stiffness and weakness and resulting in slow movement and a shuffling gait.

peer review – the rational and/or empirical scrutiny of published scientific reports by the scientific community at large.

peptide -– a molecule made up of amino acids resembling a protein, but much smaller.

peristaltic – kneading or massaging, as in the action of the esophagus when pushing food down toward the stomach.

phospholipid — any of a group of fatty compounds, composed of phosphoric esters, present in living cells (e.g. lecithin).

physiology – study of the physical and chemical processes of the cells, tissues, organs and systems of the body; the foundation of all medical science.

phytates – compounds present in some foods that affect absorption of certain vitamins or minerals.

phytonutrients – plant chemicals beneficial to human health when ingested.

pituitary gland – the 'master gland' situated in the brain that regulates and control the activity of other endocrine glands and many body processes.

placebo – an inert substance used in controlled experiments against which the efficacy of a drug is compared.

plaque – a complex deposit of lipids, platelets, calcium and scar tissue.

polyunsaturated fatty acids – any fatty acid molecule which contains more than one double bond in its carbon chain.

precursor – building block; usually simple proteins combined by the body into more complex molecules; e.g., glucose into glucosamine or beta carotene into vitamin A.

predispose – to make particularly susceptible to or inclined towards a specific response.

preventive medicine – prevention of disease states by avoiding causes or conditions under which they develop.

prognosis – probable outcome of a disease process, taking into account the effectiveness of possible therapies.

programmed cell death – apoptosis; the self-destruction of cells initiated by outside causes.

prostate cancer – a malignant growth in the outer part of the prostate gland; the most common cancer of men.

prostaglandins – one of a group of fatty acid derivatives, originally identified in human prostate secretions but now known to be present in all tissues. Different prostaglandins often have opposite actions.

prostatic hyperplasia – an overgrowth of prostate tissue.

protein – fundamental component of the body; large molecule consisting of dozens to thousands of amino acids.

proteinuria – loss of protein in the urine.

psoriasis – a chronic skin condition characterized by inflammation and scaling.

Psychosis — a severe disturbance of normal thought, perception, speech and behaviour; mental disorder involving loss of contact with reality.

quercetin – a bioflavonoid.

radiotherapy – destruction of cells by radiation targeted at cancerous cells.

reactive metabolites – toxic products of normal metabolic oxidation.

reactive oxygen molecules – reactive oxygen species; compounds containing free oxygen radicals.

receptor – a biochemical docking bay on the surface of a cell that attracts certain molecules for specific purposes and enables the cell's activity to be influenced from the outside.

relapse – re-emergence or continued advance of disease after remission.

remission – the withdrawal or temporary halt of disease and its symptoms.

reperfusion – re-established blood flow, sometimes leading to reperfusion injury.

reperfusion injury – abnormal cellular function following reperfusion.

rheumatoid arthritis – systemic arthritis caused by an auto-immune disorder.

roughage – the indigestible portion of fibrous food.

sarcoidosis – a condition of autoimmune etiology leading to inflammation and scarring of tissues throughout the body.

saturated fatty acids – a fatty acid which contains no double bonds; present in almost all fats to some degree, but highest in animal fats.

schizophrenia – a chronic, severe, and disabling brain disease often causing patients to suffer symptoms such as hearing internal voices not heard by others, or believing that other people are reading their minds, controlling their thoughts, or plotting to harm them.

scientific study – investigation or research based on scientific principles of accounting and objectivity, open to peer review.

scurvy – a disease resulting from vitamin C deficiency.

selenium – a trace element found in meat, fish, whole grains and dairy products.

sensorineural hearing loss – a problem of the inner ear or auditory nerve.

serotonin – a neurotransmitter (carries messages between nerve cells); works opposite to melatonin; serotonin is produced in response to increasing daylight to help you get out of bed in the morning.

shaking palsy – Parkinson's disease; a neurological disorder characterized by muscular tremors, stiffness and weakness and resulting in slow movement and a shuffling gait.

sinusitis – inflammation or infection of the membranes lining the sinus cavities.

SLE – systemic lupus erythematosus (lupus); chronic inflammation of the connective tissue that holds body structures together.

smooth muscle – involuntary muscle of all internal organs; usually in the form of tubes or sheets, which may be several layers in thickness.

steroids – pharmaceutical corticosteroid drugs used against disease.

stomach ulcer – also called peptic ulcers; spots where the lining of stomach has been eroded, leaving an open wound.

stress – physical, emotional, environmental or biochemical pressure.

stroke – death of or damage to brain tissue resulting from blood deprivation.

sun lamp – electrical device that simulates sunlight, including ultraviolet radiation.

sustained release – a process like *timed release*, e.g. when consuming carbohydrates high in fiber, the sugars (carbohydrates) are released more slowly than if the food consumed had no fiber.

synergistic – the mutual enhancement of separate substances by which they enhance each other's efficacy.

synergy – when the sum of two or more substances, working together, is greater, or more beneficial, than if each of those substances were working separately.

thrush – infection of the mouth or gullet by the fungus candida albicans.

tissue – a collection of cells specialized to perform a specific function.

toxicity – poisoning leading to impaired bodily function and/or cell damage.

trans fats – a fat that has been changed from its original form through either hydrogenation, heating or other type of action; usually refers to poly or monounsaturated fatty acids that have had their double bonds broken and hydrogen added.

trauma – the medical term for injury, usually referring to physical injury but also used to describe psychological injury.

tripeptide – a protein consisting of three amino acids.

tube feeding – nutrition supplied directly to the stomach or intestines.

ulcerative colitis – UC; a chronic inflammatory disease of the mucous membranes of the colon leading to ulcers.

urethral passage – the path followed by urine from the bladder to the outside of the body.

urologist – physician specializing in disorders of the urinary tract.

vascular – pertaining to blood vessels.

vasculitis – inflammation of blood vessels.

vertebrae – individual bones of the spine. **vitamins** – a group of complex nutrients not providing energy but essential in small amounts to the functioning of the body.

water-soluble – able to dissolve in water at normal temperature and pressure.

whey isolate protein – protein derived in highly pure concentrations from the liquid portion of cow's milk.

white blood cells – leukocytes (neutrophils, lymphocytes and monocytes); cells that help protect the body against disease and infection; the main components of the immune system.

whole foods – any food that hasn't undergone changes by manufacturing or processing; a food that is as close as possible to its original, natural form.

xenobiotic – substance foreign to the body and/or biological processes, including infections and toxins.

Bibliography

- Allergies, Disease in Disguise, by Carolee Bateson-Koch DC ND, *alive books*, 1994

- An Illustrated History of Medicine, by Roberto Margotta, The Hamlyn Publlishing Group, 1967

- Anesthesia, Third Edition, Edited by Ronald D. Miller, Churchill Livingstone, 1990

- Aromatherapy for Everyone, Tisserand, Robert, 1988.

- Awareness Heals, The Feldenkrais Method for Dynamic Health, by Steven Shafarman, Perseus Books, 1997

- Beyond The 120 Year Diet, by Roy Walford, M.D., Four Walls Eight Windows, 2000

- BIO-AGE Ten Steps To A Younger You, by Brad J. King and Dr. Michael A. Schmidt, Macmillan Canada, 2001

- Biochemical and Physiological Aspects of Human Nutrition, by M. Stipanuk 2000.

- Black Patent Shoes, Dancing With MS, by Eva Marsh, Sideroad Press, 1996

- Body Change by Montel Williams and Wini Linguvic, Mountain Movers Press, 2001

- Braving the Void, Journeys into Healing, by Dr. Michael Greenwood, PARADOX Publishers, 1997

- Chicken Soup for the Soul, Living Your Dreams, by Jack Canfield and Mark Victor Hansen, Health Communications, Inc., 2003

- Clinical Guide to Nutrition & Dietary Supplements in Disease Management, by Jennifer Jamison, Churchill Livingstone, 2003

- Eat Right For Your Blood Type, Dr. Peter J. d'Adamo with Catherine Whitney, G.P. Putnam's Sons, 1996

- Eating Well for Optimum Health, by Andrew Weil, M.D., Alfred A. Knoph, New York, 2000

- Essentials of Complementary and Alternative Medicine by Wayne B. Jonas, M.D. and Jeffrey S. Levin, Ph.D., M.P.H., Lippincott Williams & Wilkins, 1999

- Fats that Heal Fats that Kill, by Udo Erasmus, *alive books*, 1997

- Flaxseed in Human Nutrition, by Lilian U. Thompson and Stephen C. Cunnane, AOCS Press, 2003

- Food & Nutrition, Prevention Magazine, Edited by Feltman, John. Rodale Press, Inc. 1993

- Food, Nutrition, & Diet Therapy, by L. Kathleen Mahan and Sylvia Escott-Stump, Elsevier, 2004

- GAC Juice Ancient Fruits Modern Powerhouse, Charles C. Harpe, M.D., Sound Concepts Publishing, 2005

- Gluten-Free Diet, by Shelley Case, B.Sc., RD, Case Nutrition Consulting, 2003

- Internal Medicine, Editor-in-Chief Jay H. Stein, Little, Brown and Company, 1983

- Textbook of Medical Physiology by Arthur C. Guyton, W.B. Saunders Company, 1986

- The Oxford Medical Companion, Edited by John Walton, Jeremiah A. Barondess and Stephen Lock, Oxford University Press, 1994

- The Tufts University Guide to Total Nutrition, by Stanley Gershoff, Ph.D., Harper Perennial, 1996

- GSH, Your Body's Most Powerful Protector, GLUTATHIONE, Jimmy Gutman MD, FACEP Communications Kudo.ca Inc., Montreal, 2002

- Handbook of Clinical Nutrition and Aging, edited by C. Watkins Bales and C. Seel Ritchie, Humana Press 2004
- Hard to Swallow, by Doris Sarjeant and Karen Evans, *alive books*, 1999
- Healing Back Pain, by John E. Sarno, M.D., Warner Books, 1991
- The Healing Power of Enzymes, by DicQie Fuller, Ph.D., D.Sc.,Forbes Custom Publishing, 2002
- Healing Words, The Power of Prayer and The Practice of Medicine, by Larry Dossey, M.D., Harper, San Francisco, 1993
- Healthy Immunity, by Lorna R. Vanderhaeghe, Macmillan Canada, 2001
- Inner Vision, by Craig MacFarlane with Gib Twyman, Addax Publishing Group, 1997
- Krause's Food, Nutrition & Diet Therapy, edited by L.K. Mahan and S. Escott-Stump, Elselvier, 2004
- Laugh, I thought I'd Die, My Life with ALS, by Dennis Kaye, Penguin Books, 1994
- Law of ATTRACTION, by Michael J. Losier, Michael J. Losier, 2003
- Living with Multiple Sclerosis A Wellness Approach, by George H. Kraft, M.D. and Marci Cantanzaro, R.N., Ph.D., Demos Vermande, 1996
- Mars and Venus Together Forever, by John Gray, Ph.D., HarperPerennial, 1996
- Mind Power Into The 21st Century, by John Kehoe, Zoetic Inc, 2004
- Multiple Sclerosis, A Self-Help Guide to Its Management, by Judy Graham, Healing Arts Press, 1989
- Multiple Sclerosis, The Facts You Need, by Dr. Paul O'Connor, Key Porter Books, 1998
- Multiple Sclerosis, The Guide to Treatment and Management, Chris H. Polman, Alan J. Thompson, T. Jock Murray, W. Ian McDonald, Demos Medical Publishing, Inc., 2001

- Mutant Message From Forever, by Marlo Morgan, Harper-Perennial, 1999
- Nature's Goldmine, Harvesting Miracle Ingredients from Milk, by Allan C. Somersall, Ph.D., M.D., GOLDENeight Publishers, 2001
- Never Give Up, Crofton's Lillian Postgate at 80, by Heidi Oeste, SHALOM PRODUCTIONS, CANADA, 1999
- PDR for Nutritional Supplements, First Edition, Thomson Healthcare, Medical Economics Company, Inc, at Montvale, N.J. 2001
- Potential Within. A Guide To Nutritional Empowerment, by Franco Cavaleri, Biologic Publishing Inc., 2003
- Prescription for Nutritional Healing, James F. Balch, MD, Phyllis A. Balch, C.N.C., Avery Publishing Group, 1997
- Real Age, Are You as Young as You Can Be?, Michael F. Roizen, M.D., Realage, 1999
- Relaxercise, The Easy New Way to Health & Fitness, by David Zemach-Bersin, Kaethe Zemach-Bersin, Mark Reese, HarperSanFrancisco, 1990
- Reversing Heart Disease by Dr. Dean Ornish, Ballantine books, 1990.
- Self-Healing: My life and vision by Meir Schneider, ARKANA, The Penguin Group, 1989
- Symptom Management in Multiple Sclerosis, by Randall T. Schapiro, M.D., Demos Medical Publishing Co., Inc., 1998
- Taking Control of Multiple Sclerosis, by Professor George Jelinek, MD, Hylan House Publishing Pty Ltd, 2000
- The Antioxidant Miracle, by Lester Packer, PH.D. and Carol Colman, John Wiley & Sons, Inc. 1999
- The Antioxidant Revolution, by Dr. J.F. Balch, Sound-Concepts, 2003
- The Benefits of Nutritional Supplements, Council for Responsible Nutrition, 2002

- The China Study, by T. Colin Campbell PhD with Thomas M. Campbell II, Benbella Books, 2005
- The Food Connection by Sam Graci, Macmillan Canada, 2001
- The Fragrant Pharmacy, p. 98, Bantam Books, 1993, Valerie Ann Worwood
- The Handbook of Self-Healing, by Meir Schneider and Maureen Larkin with Dror Schneider, ARKANA Penguin Books, 1994
- The Last Taboo: A Survival Guide to Mental Health Care in Canada, by Scott Simmie and Julia Nunes, McClelland & Stewart Ltd., 2001
- The Omega-3 Phenomenon, by Donald O. Rudin, M.D., and Clara Felix with Constance Schrader, Collier Macmillan Canada, Inc., 1987
- The Origin of Medical Terms, by Henry Alan Skinner, Hafner Publishing Company, 1979
- The Pharmacology of Vitamin D, Including Fortification Strategies by R. Vieth. In Vitamin D edited by Feldman, Glorieux & Pike, 2004.
- The Power of NOW, by Eckhart Tolle, Namaste Publishing Inc., 1997
- The Probiotic Solution, Nature's Best-Kept Secret for Radiant Health, by Dr. Mark A. Brudnak, Dragon Door Publications, Inc. 2003
- The Unbroken Field. The Power of Intention in Healing, by Dr. Michael Greenwood, Paradox Publishers 2004
- Wheat-Free Cooking, by Phyllis Potts, Beyond Words Publishing, 1998
- When Your Body Gets The Blues, by Marie-Annette Brown, Ph.D., R.N., and Jo Robinson, The Berkley Publishing Group, 2003

Scientific Journals and Articles

Davis D, Epp M, Riordan H. Changes in USDA Food Composition Data for 43 Garden Crops, 1950 to 1999. Journal of the American College of Nutrition 2004; 23 (6):669-682.

Embry A. et al Vitamin D and Seasonal Fluctuations of Gadolinium-Enhancing Magnetic Resonance Imaging Lesions in Multiple Sclerosis; Annals of Neurology 2000 Aug, 48(2):271-2.

Embry A. Vitamin D Supplementation in the fight against multiple sclerosis. Personal communication.

Gillie O. Sunlight Robbery: Health benefits of sunlight are denied by current public health policy in the UK. Health Research Forum 2004. Occasional Reports: No 1.

Guggenmos J et al. Antibody cross-reactivity between myelin oligodendrocyte glycoprotein and the milk protein butyrophilin in multiple sclerosis. Journal of Immunology 2004 Jan 1; 172(1):661-8.

Heo H, Lee C. Protective effects of quercetin and vitamin C against oxidative stress – induced neurodegeneration J. Agric Food Chem. 2004; 52(25); 7514-7517.

Kennel De March A, De Bouwerie M, Kolopp-Sarda MN, Faure GC, Béné MC, Bernard CCA. Anti-myelin olegodendrocyte B-cell responses in multiple sclerosis. Journal of Neuroimmunology 135(2003) 117-125.

Linington R, Brehm U, Egg R, Dilitz E, Deisenhamme F, Poewe W, Berger L. Antibodies against the myelin oligodendrocyte glycoprotein and the myelin basic protein in multiple sclerosis and other neurological diseases: A comparative study. Brain 1999 Nov; 122(PHI):2047-56.

Liu BA, Gordon M, Labranche JM, Murray TM, Vieth R, Shear NH. Seasonal prevalence of vitamin D deficiency in institutionalized older adults. Journal of the American Geriatrics Society 1997; 45(5):598-603.

Lopez A, et al Effect of emu oil on auricular inflammation induced with croton oil in mice. American Journal of Veterinary Research; 1999 60 (12):1558-1561

Majamaa H, Isolauri E. Probiotics: a novel approach in the management of food allergy. Journarl of Allergy and Clinical Immunology 1997; Feb;99 (2):179-85.

Mana P, Goodyear M, Bernard C, Tomioka R, Freire-Garabal M, Linares D. Tolerance induction by molecular mimicry: prevention and suppression of experimental autoimmune encephalomyelitis with the milk protein butyrophilin. Int. Immunol. 2004 Mar; 16(3) 489-99.

Mather I, Jacks L. A review of the molecular and cellular biology of butyrophilin, the major protein of bovine milk fat globule membrane. Journal of Dairy Science 1992.

Mathey E, Breithaupt C, Schubart A, Linington C. Sorting the wheat from the chaff: identifying demyelinating components of the myelin oligodendrocyte glycoprotein (MOG)-specific autoantibody repertoire. Eur. J. Immunol. 2004, 34: 2065-2071.

Moongkarndi, P et al Antiproliferative activity of Thai medicinal plant extracts on human breast adenocarcinoma cell line. Fitoterapia 2004; 75:375-377.

Nakatani K et al. Inhibitions of histamine release and prostaglandin E_2 synthesis by mangosteen, a Thai medicinal plant. Biol Pharm Bull 2002; 25(9); 1137-1141.

Nakatani K, et al. Kuni T, Kondo N, Arakawa. Gamma mangostin inhibits inhibitor KB Kinase activity and decreases Lipopolysaccharide-Induced Cyclooxygenase-2 Gene Expression in C6 Rat Glioma Cells. Mol Pharmacol 66:667-674. 2004.

Ogg SL, Weldon AK, Dobbie L, Smith AJ, Mather IH. Expression of butyrophilin (BTN 1a1) in lactating mammary gland is essential for the regulated secretion of milk-lipid droplets. Proc Natl Acad Sci USA 2004 Jul 6; 101(27): 10084-9.

Omega 3 Fatty Acids and their Impact on Cardiovascular Disease, Triglycerides, and Anti Inflammatory Actions. Presented by Dr. B. Holub, Department of Human Biology and Nutritional Sciences, University of Guelph, November 26, 2004.

Politis MJ, Dmytrowich A. Promotion of Second Intention Wound healing by emu oil lotion. Comparative results with furasin, polysporin and cortisone Plast. Reconstr. Surg. 1998;102: 2404-2407.

Reindl, M et al Antibodies against the myelin oligodendrocyte glycoprotein and the myelin basic protein in multiple sclerosis and other neurological diseases: a comparative study. Brain 1999; 122:2047-2056.

Rosbo K et al. Predominance of the autoimmune response to myelin oligodendrocyte glycoprotein (MOG) in multiple sclerosis: reactivity to the extracellular domain of MOG is directed against three main regions Eur J Immunol. 1997 Nov; 27(11): 3059-69.

Snowden JM, Whitehouse MW. Anti-inflammatory activity of emu oil in rats. Inflammopharmacology 1997; 5:127-132.

Stefferl A et al. Butyrophilin, a milk protein, modulates the encephalitogenic T cell response to myelin oligodendrocyte glycoprotein in experimental autoimmune encephalomyelitis. J Immunol. 2000 Sept 1; 165(5): 2859-65.

Trang HM, Cole DE, Rubin LA, Pierratos A, Siu S, Vieth R. Evidence that vitamin D_3 increases serum 25-hydroxyvitamin D more efficiently than does vitamin D_2. Am J. Clin. Nutr. 1998; 68(4):854-8.

Van der Aa A, Hellings N, Bernard CC, Rous J, Stinssen P. Functional properties of myelin oligodendrocyte glycoprotein – reactive T cells in multiple sclerosis of patients and controls. J Neuroimmunol. 2003; 137(1-2): 164-176.

Van der Mei I, Ponsonby A, Blizzard L, Dwyer T. Regional variation in Multiple Sclerosis prevalence in Australia and its association with ambient Ultraviolet radiation. Neuroepidemiology 2001 Aug; 20(3):168-74.

Vieth R, Chan Pak-Cheung R, MacFarlane G. Efficacy and safety of vitamin D_3 intake exceeding the lowest observed adverse effect level. Am J Clin Nutr 2001; 73: 288-94.

Vieth R. Vitamin D nutrition and its potential health benefits for bone, cancer and other conditions. J. Envir. and Nut. Med.. 2001; 11(4):1-12.

Weissert R, et al. High immunogenicity of intracellular myelin oligodendrocyte glycoprotein epitopes. J Immunol. 2002 July 1; 169(1):548-56.

Resources

EMU Consulting Corp.
Box 877
Duncan, B.C. Canada V9L 3Y2
Phone: 1-888-784-2244
Fax: 1-250-746-4803
Website: www.drbillcode.com
Email: info@drbillcode.com

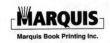

Marquis Book Printing Inc.

Québec, Canada
2008